Great
Skin
—for life

Karen Burke *M.D., Ph.D.*

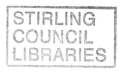

HAMLYN

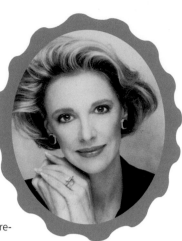

Karen Burke is a dermatologist and research scientist with a Ph.D. in biophysics from Cornell University and an M.D. from New York University. She is in private practice in New York City where she is also a Staff Member at Cabrini Medical Center. Dr. Burke is known for her research on the prevention and reversal of aging of the skin as well as the prevention and treatment of skin cancer and has published research papers on many subjects, including fat structure and metabolism. She is a foremost authority in the field of cosmetic dermatology, and a frequent consultant to both pharmaceutical and cosmetic companies. Because she believes that "the best cosmetic of all is naturally healthy skin", she has researched and formulated her own exclusive line of Longévité® skincare products. Dr. Burke has written numerous articles and is frequently quoted as a health and skincare expert in magazines such as *Vogue*, *Harper's Bazaar*, *Glamour*, *Elle* and *Family Circle*. She is author of *Thin Thighs for Life* – the first book in her popular "Great Health for Life" series. Dr. Burke has also made numerous television and radio appearances in the USA, Great Britain, France and Germany. She is married and lives in New York.

Author's Acknowledgments

With my special thanks to my husband Peter and to Heather Nolan, Patricia H. Page and Franklin J. Wright Ph D; and with great appreciation to my mentors in dermatology and medicine Rudolf L. Baer M.D., A. Bernard Ackerman M.D., Alfred W. Kopf M.D., George L. Popkin M.D., Gloria F. Graham M.D., Louie L. Patseavou... M.D. and Robert M. Makamura M.D.

Commissioning Editor: Jane McIntosh
Art Director: Keith Martin
Senior Designer: Ben Barrett
Designer: Paul Webb
Editors: Mary Lambert, Anne Johnson
Picture Research: Jenny Faithfull
Production Controller: Melanie Frantz
Illustrator: Vicky Emptage

First published in Great Britain in 1996 by Hamlyn, an imprint of Reed International Books Limited
Michelin House, 81 Fulham Road, London SW3 6RB
and Auckland, Melbourne, Singapore and Toronto

Text © Karen Burke
Illustrations and design © Reed International Books Limited

ISBN 0 600 58989 7

Produced by Mandarin Offset
Printed in Hong Kong

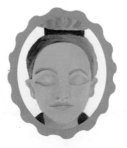

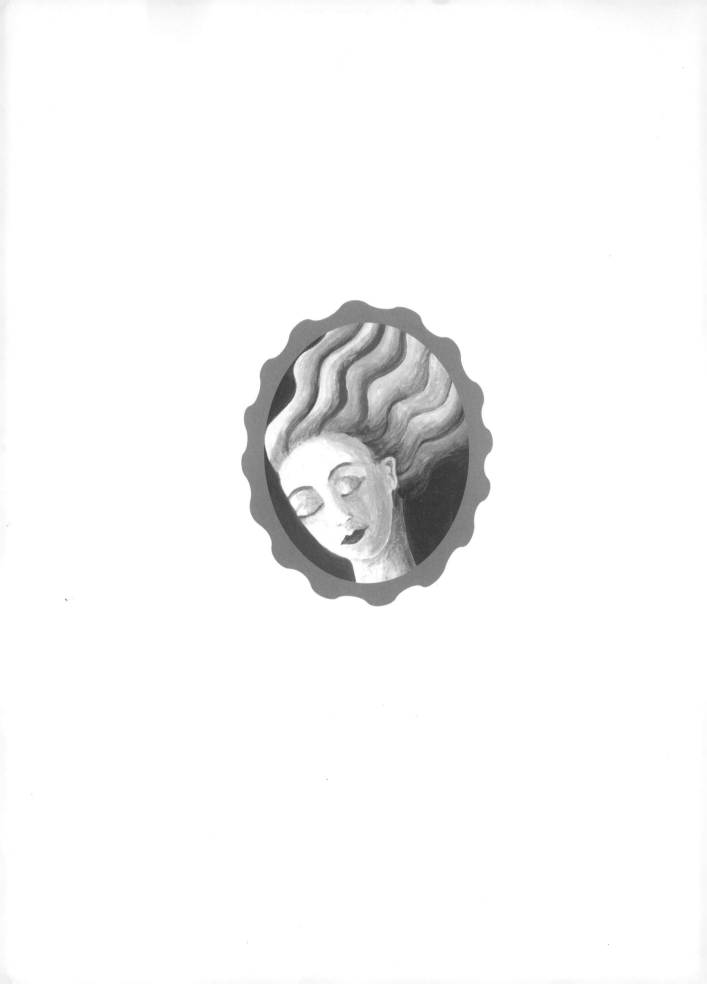

Contents

Foreword

The skin is your body's sheath, your protection and your "calling card", the subtle but important signal you project to the world about who you are and what you are made of. I have come to realize that skincare is a truly marvellous pursuit, richly rewarded by the joy of a younger and finer appearance, and by improved health!

Having dedicated my career in science and dermatology to studying the science and medicine of the skin, I share daily with my friends and patients the secrets of excellent skincare. In the pages of this book, I gladly share all these secrets with you.

Twenty-five years ago, the science of the skin was much less advanced. Although at that time dermatologists knew how to effectively treat skin problems, they did not necessarily understand precisely how or why their remedies actually worked. Nor did scientists focus their research on understanding the skin's normal aging process or the effects that the environment had on the natural aging process.

Today, as a consequence of recent and rapid scientific advances, a lot more is understood about these processes, and progress is being made in how to delay and even reverse them. Yes ... reverse the aging of the skin! Through the pages of this book, I will convey to you some of this knowledge in terms everyone can understand. The "wonders" of science, coupled with common sense, really can and will do wonders for your skin.

When you read a magazine or you enter a department store today, you are confronted by hundreds of different skincare products and thousands of conflicting claims and promises. You are promised or sold, as the saying goes, "hope in a bottle". Some of the claims may be accurate and some of the products may work quite well. But how are you to judge what is really best for you?

Great Skin For Life will be your guide. You will learn about your skin. No matter what your environment, what your skin problems or your ethnic

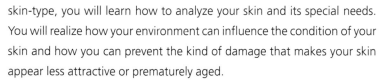

"How I love to contemplate the brilliance of your skin,
shimmering fabric reflecting your beautiful body."
Baudelaire

skin-type, you will learn how to analyze your skin and its special needs. You will realize how your environment can influence the condition of your skin and how you can prevent the kind of damage that makes your skin appear less attractive or prematurely aged.

By simply avoiding sun exposure and tanning salons, you can look decades younger later in life! As you will see, common problems such as dry skin, rashes, and even acne can be caused or worsened by your indoor environment. With understanding, you can often eliminate many of the causes of your skin problems.

Now that we can all expect to enjoy healthier and more active lives for far longer than any generation before us, we can also all "look as young as we feel". As you will learn, skincare that shows wonderful and lasting results need be neither difficult, nor time-consuming, nor expensive. *Great Skin For Life* gives a personalized programme of skincare that is not only comprehensive but that also really works, for men as well as for women!

In researching and developing my own line of Longévité® skincare products, I adopted the maxim: "Beauty is health and health is beauty", along with the phrase, "The best cosmetic of all is naturally healthy skin". I am completely dedicated to this philosophy and I'm genuinely delighted to share with you in the pages that follow the knowledge that will help you attain, and maintain, great skin ... for life.

*NOTE: **Great Skin for Life** provides useful information about the skin. It does not consti-tute or contain medical advice, and it is not a substitute for regular check-ups or periodic visits to your doctor or dermatologist. If you have any reason to believe that you have a condition requiring medical treatment, you should see your doctor immediately. Even if you are not aware of any specific problems, this might be a good time to have a complete medical and dermatological examination.*

The Story of Skin

The science is new. The custom is not! Modern skincare is part of a continuing practice that is older than the human race. Skin grooming is a
practice inherited from our pre-historic ancestors (as a trip to the zoo or a
look at your cat will confirm!). Skin adornment, on the other hand, is
distinct to "human" cultures throughout history – a trait that sets us apart
from other animals.

Skincare and the cosmetic enhancement of the skin are part of the rich panorama of history, which is linked inextricably to conquests, geographic exploration, trade, cultural exchange, social custom, religion, philosophy, moral codes, scientific discovery and art. In the Paleolithic age, skincare might have meant applying protective animal grease; in later primitive societies it was a daub of war paint; to the Egyptians it was a perfumed body oil; to the Elizabethans it was a facial mask; and to the "modern woman" it is a quick shower and a touch of lipstick and mascara. Human skin was the first organ to be cared for, and the first canvas to be painted.

Cave care

Over a million years ago Paleolithic men and women rubbed animal fat on their bodies, not for "looks" but to protect themselves from the elements. They used red ochre powder (from iron ore found in stone) for healing. By 100,000 BC, Neanderthal hunters painted their bodies for camouflage. They and their descendants, Stone Age man, also practised the first purely "cosmetic" skin adornment – tattooing – whether as custom or possibly to terrify aggressors. The practice survived to our day. The tribesmen of Melanesia, for example, engendered fear by painting their ribs with white clay to resemble living skeletons.

As "civilization" progressed with its spirituality and ritual, man deified the forces of nature in ceremonies in which they painted body and face with animal likenesses, "transferring" the beast's strength to the bearer. These markings later served as tribal identification, and symbols of status within the tribe. Stages of life were also symbolized by the decoration of skin and hair. Puberty was celebrated with rituals including painting the body, plucking hair, tattooing, and cutting or burning to "decorate" with scars. Enduring pain was part of the initiation. The erroneous concept, "suffering achieves beauty", still in vogue today, may come from these primitive ceremonies in which adulthood was first earned through rough "cosmetic injury".

In the shadow of the pyramids

Thanks to their view of the after-world (and what they needed to take along!), the Egyptians were entombed complete with their clothing and cosmetics so that they were ready to embark on their after-life in style. Skincare and cosmetics achieved their first "golden age" in the Egyptian world, dating from as early as 4000 BC.

The Egyptians had an extraordinary understanding of personal hygiene: daily bathing for health and pleasure was common practice, unlike other ancient societies in which bathing was limited to religious ceremonies. As documented in the *Ebero Papyrus* (the oldest known medical document, c. 1500 BC), the Egyptians invented a soap-like material used for treating skin diseases and washing. Oils and ointments to protect from sand, dust, and dryness were not luxuries, but much prized necessities used throughout society. During the reign of Ramses III, the gravediggers of Thebes actually went on strike to protest a decline in the quality of their food and the quantity of their oils! And Pharaoh Sete I reinforced the loyalty of his army by increasing their allocation of ointments.

The timeless elegance of Queen Nefertiti and the regal distinction of King Tut-Ankh-Amon, with eyes so dramatically outlined, are among the most striking images of all time. The eye, the symbol of the Sun God Ra, was the Egyptians' most cosmetically accentuated feature. Men, children and women applied eyeliner of black lead or silver nitrate and eye shadow of green malachite or blue azurite derived from copper ores. This eye "makeup" was more than cosmetic; it reduced glare, kept away insects, and helped fight infections, especially the dreaded "river blindness". (Silver nitrate is still today dropped into the eyes of newborns to prevent infection.) For special occasions the Egyptians added a decorative "eye glitter" of crushed, iridescent beetle-shells. (The "punk" look is older than you thought!)

Egyptian women applied fat or oil tinged with red ochre to their lips and cheeks to moisturize and to add colour. They reddened their palms and fingernails with henna dye, accentuated the veins in their temples and breasts with blue pigment, and gilded their nipples with gold paint! They also, however, initiated a practice that was to harm skin for centuries: whitening the face with dangerous lead foundations.

Men applied as much makeup as women, adding orange ochre flesh tone to appear sunburned and masculine. Egyptian recipes for

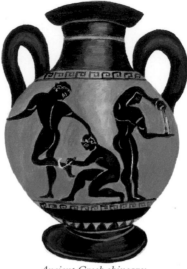

Ancient Greek skincare: athletes cleaned themselves with aromatic oils which were removed with a strigil.

animal- or vegetable-based protective ointments scented with flower petals or spices have survived to the present day. Queen Cleopatra herself left us a treatise on beauty preparations, including potions for smoothing the skin and treating blemishes and a dubious cure for baldness which contained arsenic!

The Egyptians exported their cosmetics and scented unguents throughout the ancient world: toiletries were so commonly used by the Hebrews' Second Temple Period that the Talmud advised husbands to allocate ten dinars for their wives' cosmetic needs.

Greek refinement

Classical Greek skincare, influenced by the importance of sport, differed markedly from that of the Egyptians. By the 4th century BC, Greek palaestras and gymnasia were equipped with elaborate baths. With modern soap not yet invented, the Greeks cleansed their bodies with blocks of clay, sand, pumice and ashes. Before a competition, athletes oiled their skin, sprinkled on powder, and then later removed the mixture with a metal scraper, a *strigil*, so often depicted in Greek painting and pottery. Bathing and anointing the body with aromatic oils and perfumes were essential to daily routine. In fact by the 2nd century BC, bathrooms were a regular fixture in homes, even of the middle classes.

The classical Greek aesthetic is characterized by simplicity and elegance – in art, architecture, philosophy and fashion. Although the word "cosmetic" stems from the Greek *kosmetikos* (meaning "skilled in decoration"), Greek wives used cosmetics sparingly in their male-dominated society. Notwithstanding the powerful and beautiful women of Homeric and Olympic legend, Greek women held astonishingly limited social positions, with housewives confined to segregated quarters. A Greek wife's application of even minimal color to her cheeks or lips made her husband suspect her of adultery.

Not so with the Greek courtesans, the *hetaerae* whose seductive skills called for lavish makeup. These women, the "geishas" of classical Greece, gave up matrimony for an education in poetry, music, dance, and even philosophy. By no means prostitutes; they were highly sought after and even respected. Men lavished them with gifts, and Pindar, the great poet himself, composed an ode to their attraction.

The rising sun

The great civilizations of the Far East – China, Japan, southeast Asia and the Indian sub-continent – also have their own great and ancient traditions of skincare and makeup. In many instances, makeup and markings had much more than cosmetic significance, indicating the wearer's role as well as social status. Alexander the Great reached India and the borders of China, and the earliest trade routes brought much-prized eastern fragrances and oils to the west, a continuing influence on western practices and customs.

The Roman bath

The Romans eagerly incorporated Greek culture and practice, including hygiene, skincare, and cosmetics. As Roman civilization spread with their conquests, so did bathing. Bathing was a social occasion central to everyday Roman life. With aqueducts to supply water, luxurious public baths became widely accessible, each with a *tepidarium* (warm room), a *caldarium* (hot room), and a *frigidarium* (cold room), and rooms for massage. The Romans selected special ointments for each part of the body and women kept their valuable unguents with them in a locked box.

Along with the elevation of bathing to an art, the Romans made two contributions to skincare appreciated to this day – soap and cold cream. With the sacrifice of animals to the gods, rain washed the resulting mixture of melted animal fat and wood ash into soil along the Tiber River. Women discovered that this clay effectively washed their clothes and themselves, and (fortunately for us!) their chemists attributed this phenomenon to more than the holiness of the waters. The Romans' place of animal sacrifice was called *Mount Sapo*, hence the word "soap"!

Galen, a 2nd century Roman and skincare guru, was chief physician to the school of gladiators and to the imperial family. He formulated medications against infection and also devised beauty aids for patrician women. One of his creations, cold cream, safely and effectively softened and cleansed the skin with a mixture of wax, olive oil and rosewater. Galen was also the first to recommend oil (lanolin) from sheep's wool as a moisturizer.

Rome set new standards in hygiene and

cosmetic care, which are impressive to this day! Men and women brushed their teeth, tweezed their eyebrows, curled their hair, and cared for their faces by applying overnight face packs with original, and often unappetizing, ingredients such as sheep fat and crocodile excrement! Pippaea, Nero's wife, used alpha hydroxy acids to eliminate wrinkles, travelling with a herd of goats to bathe in their milk (rich in lactic acid).

Cosmetic art was highly developed. Women painted their faces and arms with white lead powder; rouged their lips and cheeks with red ochre, and darkened their eyebrows and lashes with kohl or burnt cork; men also applied makeup. Ovid, himself the inventor of ointments giving "shining" white complexions, criticized Roman women for an excess of cosmetic artifice, advising that: *"The art that adorns you should be unsuspected."*

Celts, Dark Ages, Crusaders

Dressed in animal skins, the nomadic Celts of Britain were civilized only minimally by the Druids, whose witchcraft and knowledge of herbs introduced ointments with "magical powers" to cure wounds or enhance beauty. With Roman occupation the Celts adopted Roman practices. The elaborate designs with which they painted their bodies were transferred to their shields, evolving later into coats-of-arms. With the invasion of tattooed Germanic barbarians and the decline of Roman civilization, "dark ages" were in store for skincare. The spread of Christianity brought a rejection of bathing as ungodly vanity, and then unsanitary conditions contributed to the Black Death of the 14th

century and the other great plagues of the Middle Ages. Contributions to skincare were limited to hand-cream formulations.

With the Crusades, Europeans were extremely impressed with the silks, spices, carpets, pillows, birds, ornaments, baths with luxuriant oils, cosmetics and perfumes that were the opulence and refinement of the East. Many Crusaders stayed to enjoy them; others brought these Eastern influences home.

The French in particular developed elaborate cosmetic preparations such as powder, rouge, and hair colorants made from plants and wine rather than lead and arsenic. Italy, Spain and France became centres of soap making using olive oil. Unfortunately, English women were still restrained from the "artificial vanities" of skincare and hygiene by a Puritan ethic which punished any practice of such "devil's evil".

The skincare renaissance

The Renaissance revived an appreciation of cosmetic care, beginning in Italy and reaching England in the 16th century reign of Elizabeth I. Elizabeth, obsessed with preserving her looks, adopted the liberal use of cosmetics, applying white powder and rouge made from lead (the ingredient so damaging to women's skin over the centuries) or ground alabaster, colorful eye shadows, and even makeup for the hands and tints for the teeth! White skin was so admired that women wore masks (kept in place by buttons held in their teeth) and perfumed gloves to protect their skin from the sun. The first sunscreens were developed at this time from thin glazes of egg-white.

As she aged, Elizabeth painted artificial veins on her forehead and breasts to simulate a youthful, translucent complexion, and invented recipes for facial masks containing milk and wine to tighten wrinkles and sulfur to help her reddish complexion. She liberally applied perfumed moisturizing oils, but resorted to a "drastic bath" only once a month!

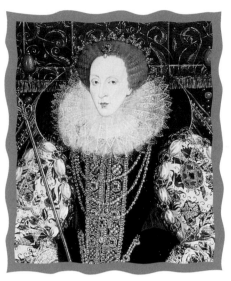

Queen Elizabeth I looked after her empire, but she still found time to take care of her skin.

Cosmetics versus the Puritans

The two centuries following Elizabeth's reign saw the legacy of Elizabethan cosmetics (influenced by Parisian society) do battle with Puritan restrictions. Men and women continued to spend time and money on their *toilette*, women liberally applying dreadful white lead powder and rouge to their cheeks and lips. "Beauty patches" of black silk or velvet were worn over smallpox scars. The Puritans opposed any such "artifice": a high tax was levied on soap and Cromwell unsuccessfully backed a Parliamentary act against the "Vice of Painting and Wearing Black Patches".

As late as 1770, legislation to the effect that "women ... who seduce or betray into matrimony, by scents, paint, or cosmetic washes ... shall incur the penalty of the law as against witchcraft, and that marriage shall stand null and void" was proposed and defeated.

Despite the Puritans, frivolity and cosmetics flourished, as can be seen in the elaborate makeup and powdered curls of Gainsborough's portraits of society's beauties. Remarkably, lead was still a principal ingredient despite the obvious illness of manufacturers and users. Opulence was on the rise, influenced especially by the French court: Marie Antoinette spent most of her waking hours pursuing her skincare and cosmetic regimen, including bathing in red wine! This increasing extravagance came to a halt with the French Revolution. The English retired to the countryside, and makeup went "out" of fashion.

A clean body

In Europe during the 1800s, the 6,000-year-old cosmetic staples – perfume, oils, rouge, facial powder, and lipstick – almost disappeared. With the rejection of artifice came a new approach to skincare, one followed by today's dermatologists: improving the natural condition of the skin rather than camouflaging its faults. Cleanliness and sun protection were paramount. An unwashed body masked by heavy perfume or dirty hair disguised with powder was no longer acceptable. Products to *treat* the skin (moisturizers, sunscreens, bleaches for freckles) were homemade following recipes described in *The Art of Beauty*, an influential book anonymously published in France in 1825. Included were formulations for subtle makeup based on plants, containing none of the toxic ingredients of previous ages.

By Queen Victoria's reign, daily baths had once again become routine, the heavy tax on soap was lifted, and soap making was advanced by the Belgian chemist Solvay, who used soda ash to make soap inexpensive and readily available. Its manufacture and purchase thrived, especially in England and America.

The Victorian era constricted women, both figuratively and (with tightly corseted fashion) literally. Men used cosmetics quite openly, but they were forbidden to women. Across the channel, Paris was giddy with the spirit and cosmetic artifice of *la belle époque*. Books abounded with beauty secrets, describing powder made from pearls, eye shadow using paste of cloves or charcoal, and mascara mixing China ink with rosewater. Spanish women slept in gloves lined with beautifying pomade. (Dermatologists today recommend similar treatment for hands.)

Back to color

Influenced by the high fashion of Paris and by prominent actresses such as Sarah Bernhardt and Lily Langtry, the turn of the century saw the lifting of restraints on women, who again added rouge, eye shadow, and mascara to their skin regime. By the early 1900s, artifice was once again "in". Helena Rubenstein, having studied medicine in her native Poland, moved to Australia where she observed the deplorable condition of women's skin. She made available skin creams she had created for herself. Inspired by theatrical makeup, she replaced chalk-white "rice powder" with pink powder to give a natural, healthy blush, and she devised makeup to contour the face. Dramatic makeup for Sergei Diaghilev's *Ballets Russes* fuelled the rage for brightly colored cosmetics, especially eye shadows, which are enjoyed to this day.

The early 20th century gave birth to the modern cosmetics industry: Brand-name products became available to everyone by mail order or in stores. First the French, then the Americans took the lead. Avon was founded by a book salesman who realized he could sell more beauty products than Bibles!

With the First World War, women left the house to work in factories and charities, and by the "Roaring 20's" the demand for cosmetics had grown rapidly. The chemical factories of France, Germany, and the United States converted to peacetime pursuits, including the production of skincare products.

The Coco tan

Between the wars, France led the fashion world, and Coco Chanel spearheaded the (medically regrettable) craze of suntanning when her tanned models suggested the luxury of the Riviera. It has taken 60 years and millions of skin cancers to challenge this misdirected vogue.

"Glamor" became the byword of Hollywood, with silent movie stars such as Mary Pickford and Lillian Gish followed by the magnificent cosmetic "makeovers" of Garbo and Dietrich. Beauty became a popular asset for attaining a job or "the right man". The beauty salon grew into a skincare sanctuary, cosmetics became necessities.

Even during the Second World War, women spent limited funds on makeup rather than food. Lipstick was in such short supply that a survey of Navy nurses evacuated by submarines found that lipstick was the item they most often took with them! Though supplies of toiletries were rationed as companies contributed to the war effort, sales of cosmetics rose. Hollywood churned out heroic films with glamorous women (Hedy Lamarr, Rita Hayworth, Lana Turner) – all made-up to the hilt!

Modern times

Postwar skincare evolved into "big business". Competition for mass markets was fierce, and companies turned to psychologists, sociologists, and market researchers to direct consumers' desires. Advertising promised much. It was either suggested by name (Joran's *Wrinkles-Away*, Lauder's *Youth Dew*) or by flawlessly glamorous models photographed in exotic locations.

The women of the prosperous 50s were torn between two stereotypes: the pristine "girl next door" (Sandra Dee, Debbie Reynolds) or the glamorous seductress (Marilyn Monroe). The emphasis was on cover-up, not skincare.

The 60s brought social upheaval, the Beatles, the miniskirt, the civil rights movement, Vietnam and protesting students. Baby-boomers shunned "the establishment" to revel in their individuality. Top models like Lauren Hutton were not flawless, makeup was less structured and less fashionable, but true "skincare" had not yet "arrived".

The anti-establishment trends of the 60s evolved into environmentally inspired health-consciousness. By the 70s, the image of beauty became health, natural vitality, and fitness, not artifice. In 1974, for the first time in many years toiletry sales lagged behind the growth in personal spending. The public began to distrust advertising claims and to associate cosmetics with artificiality and with skin irritations, acne or more serious reactions. In an age of science and technology, the public wanted a different kind of skincare product.

New technology

Science has addressed the public's demand for safe, natural and effective skincare and cosmetics, and the best is yet to come! Today details of the skin's physiology are understood and efficacy of treatment can be measured. Through cosmetic chemistry research, pure natural ingredients are isolated and new ones are synthesized. Since the 80s, packages display the components of skincare products, deflating the hype and allowing the consumer to avoid potential irritants.

In recent years, sales of truly helpful skincare products have grown beyond all expectation. It has come full circle. Just as the "cosmetics" of primitive man and ancient civilizations were protective, so this is again a primary motivation. With everyone's realization of the dangers of sun exposure, sunscreen sales have soared. "Cosmeceuticals" – a new generation of skincare products of proven effectiveness (see Chapter 9) – are available, and everyone can be specifically treated. There is no longer a stereotypical beauty, but rather an exuberant individuality: all ethnic groups, all "looks" are "in" as long as they are healthy. Today, a *Great Skin For Life* can be achieved through knowledge and easy-to-understand science. That's what this book is all about!

Skin Science

Most of us take skin for granted and never really think about all the things it does for us. Your skin conveys your outward appearance to yourself and to the world: it's your "presentation package". But the skin is in fact a living organ – the largest organ of your body and a quite remarkable one. Skin makes up about 15 percent of your body's total weight and it covers more than 18sq ft (1.7sq miles) of surface, with the remarkable ability to stretch if you gain weight and contract when you slim down.

The skin is the only body organ that can be seen. Indeed, your skin may reveal more to the world than you might wish. It can give away your approximate age, your state of health and the way you take care of yourself. And because even the smallest skin abnormality can be immediately seen, more skin diseases are specifically named and recognized than those of any other organ.

Learning begins with touching. In our embryonic growth the skin is the first organ to form, and touch is the first sensation to develop. When an embryo which is less than 1in (25mm) long and only six weeks old (before its eyes or ears are formed) is touched, it turns to seek the source of its external stimulation.

Not only is the skin the first sensory organ, but it is also the body's most important sensory organ. If you think of people like Helen Keller and of others who have lived their lives deaf and blind, their primary communication with the world was through skin stimulation. When other senses fail, the skin compensates to an extraordinary degree. A human being can live without sight, hearing, smell and taste, but cannot survive without the sensory input of the skin.

The skin (except the lining of the stomach and intestines) is the organ which renews itself the most rapidly. In fact, the very symbol of medicine, the *caduceus* – a staff around which two serpents are entwined – held by the ancient Greek father of medicine, Asklepios, represents the curing and renewal of the body, just as the snake periodically sheds and renews its skin.

To make best use of the secrets of skincare you are about to learn from *Great Skin For Life*, you must know a bit about the astounding way in which the skin is put together and how the skin system works. To put it simply, to help your skin, you must learn how it helps you!

Your skin helps you every day

In the past you have probably marvelled at your heart as it pumps blood around your body year after year, and been thankful for your eyes as they translate light into electrical stimuli, opening a marvellous sensory window. Your skin is the largely unsung hero of your constitution. It's your first line of defence, protecting your internal organs from the external world. It also protects them from mechanical injury, from foreign substances, including infectious organisms. Your skin even has its own immune system protecting you against irritants and invading viruses, bacteria, parasites, and fungi.

Your skin is your thermostat, regulating your body's temperature through sensitive, specialized thermoreceptor cells. When skin feels heat, it reacts by stimulating sweating to cool the body. When skin feels cold, it reacts by contracting the tiny muscles around each hair follicle to induce shivering, thereby "exercising" (and burning lots of calories) to warm the body.

Skin is covered with many specialized nerves and touch receptors, each of which receives and transmits a specific sensation: pain, temperature, itching, or the size, shape and texture of objects. Through the skin, you can detect tiny temperature changes and perceive objects as small as a grain of sand or as delicate as a wisp of cotton. And through the skin you react to the most minute pain and can enjoy the ultimate pleasure.

The skin is a trader – an exchange organ –

helping to export waste products from your body and import nutrients. More and more now, modern medicine uses the skin's "absorption system" for the controlled and dependable delivery of medicines such as hormones and cardiac medications and of drugs such as nicotine to decrease smoking or scopolamine to prevent movement sickness.

Finally, your skin regulates your body's fluid balance and synthesizes vitamins, storing nutrients and medications and converting them to the forms that are required.

In short, your skin is essential not only to your good looks, but to maintain life itself! Take a look at your skin: it's a valuable friend well worth caring for.

The structure of your skin

The structure of skin, its form and its function, is amazing – a marvel of practical engineering. As you can see in the illustration opposite, the skin has two layers: the *epidermis* – the outer layer which is directly visible, the main function of which is to protect the body by forming a sheath or "carapace" of dead cells on the surface; and the *dermis,* the deeper layer which supports and nourishes the epidermis by containing not only the important structural proteins collagen and elastin, but blood vessels, nerves, hair follicles, sebaceous glands, and the sweat glands.

All over the body (except the upper eyelids, the scalp, the earlobes, the palms of the hands, the soles of the feet, the penis and the scrotum), the epidermis and dermis sit on a layer of *subcutaneous* fat. For example, if you pinch the skin on the back of your hand, that's what pure skin feels like. A "pinch test" can also tell you about the condition of your elastic tissue.

The epidermis

Your epidermis consists of about 15–25 layers of closely connected cells in four distinct layers (see illustration opposite). The epidermis varies in thickness in different parts of the body according to its functional need. It is at its thinnest on the upper eyelid where you need only a delicate protective cover that does not put pressure on the eye, and it is at its thickest on the soles of the feet where you require that extra toughness.

Skin cells are formed in the inner, or "basal", layer of the epidermis (the *stratum germinativum*). Since there is no direct blood supply in the epidermis, this basal layer needs to be just above the skin's deeper layer, the *dermis*, to benefit from the nourishment and oxygen-exchange from the dermis that is needed for the metabolism.

The cells of this basal layer are very busy, constantly reproducing to form new cells which move upward and outward toward the skin surface. As each new layer of cells forms, it displaces the overlying layer. In fact the three upper layers of the epidermis are entirely replaced about every three to four weeks! This continuous reproduction gives your skin the ability to heal well after injury, to peel after sunburn, and to rejuvenate each day with proper care.

Your skin cells don't live too long. As the epidermal cells move from the basal layer to the second layer, the *stratum spinosum* (named because the cells have distinct connections joining each to its neighbors), they begin to die. By

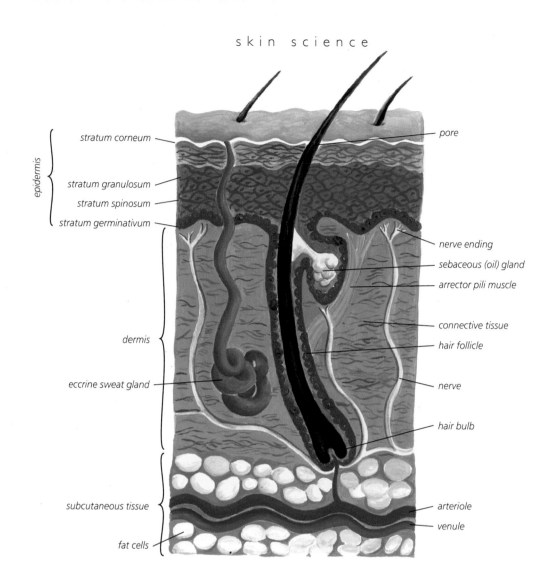

epidermis

stratum corneum

stratum granulosum

stratum spinosum

stratum germinativum

dermis

eccrine sweat gland

subcutaneous tissue

fat cells

pore

nerve ending

sebaceous (oil) gland

arrector pili muscle

connective tissue

hair follicle

nerve

hair bulb

arteriole

venule

the time they reach the third layer, the *stratum granulosum*, they are flattened, and granules consisting of *keratin* (the structural protein within skin cells) are prominent. Finally, the skin cells complete their month-long journey of migration to the skin surface, the *stratum corneum*. In contrast to the cells in the basal layer which are plump and moist (with about 80 percent water), the surface cells are dry (containing only 20 percent water, the rest keratin protein) and flat, overlapping in layers like shingles of a roof to form a strong, protective shield.

As you age, your skin is put through a rough regime. It is exposed to: sun, dry indoor environ-ments with excessive heat in winter and air conditioning in summer, pollutants like cigarette smoke, car exhaust, and solvents from building materials or freshly made fabric. Our skin rises to the defence, protecting us by creating a thicker outer level of dry skin, the dead skin of the stra-tum corneum on the surface, purposefully "glued on" to serve as a barrier, protecting the deeper layers of our skin and body.

What gives us our color?

There are other important cells in the skin's epidermal layer. About one in every ten basal cells is a *melanocyte*, the cell that produces the

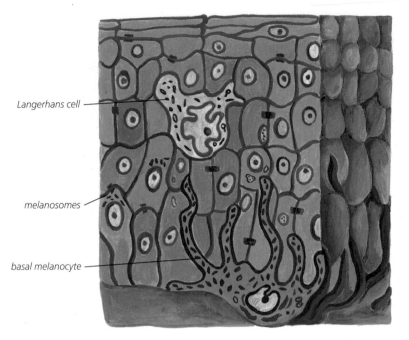

Langerhans cell

melanosomes

basal melanocyte

Transferring color to your skin: the epidermal melanin unit
Adapted from Quevedo W.C. Jr., "The Control of Color in Mammals", American Zoology 9: 531 – 540, 1969

pigment *melanin.* These cells develop from nerve tissue, and move to the skin early in embryonic development. Within the melanocyte cell, melanin (actually *eumelanin,* the brown to black pigment) or *pheomelanin* (the yellow-red pigment of the Celtic races) is synthesized, or "manufactured", by a specific enzyme. This pigment is packaged in small membrane sacks to form *melanosomes,* then it is transferred to the skin cells through the long, spider-like projections of the melanocyte (see illustration above). The average density of melanocytes varies depending upon the area of the body as shown in the illustration on page 22, but this density is about the same in all races.

The different pigmentation of the white, black, yellow, and red races is due to the way in which the pigment is packaged in the melanosome. In a Caucasian, the melanosomes are grouped together in membrane-bound melanosome complexes. The complexes also contain some small particles of pigment as well as other so-called *ground substance* (about which you will learn shortly). A very light-skinned individual with blue eyes, for example, has less pigment within each melanosome and fewer melanosome complexes in each skin cell. (A red-head also has pheomelanin instead of eumelanin within the melanosomes.) The Mongoloid – either a yellow-skinned Oriental or a red-skinned American Indian – has melanosome complexes which are smaller but much more densely packed. In Negroid skin, the melanosomes are individually dispersed and are much larger and more densely filled with pigment than those of a Caucasian or Mongoloid (see illustration opposite).

When a person of any race is exposed to the sun: 1) more melanin is synthesized; 2) more

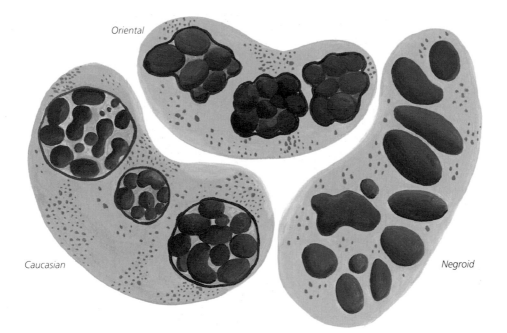

Melanosome complexes in stratum granulosum cells of three races.
Adapted from Szabó G., Gerald A.B., Pathak M.A., Fitzpatrick T.B., "Racial differences in the fate of melanosomes in human epidermis",
Nature 222: 1081–1082, 1969

melanosomes form; and 3) these melanosomes (in Blacks) or melanosome-complexes (in Whites, Orientals and Indians) are transferred in increasing numbers to neighboring skin cells, temporarily darkening the skin to a "tan". Lighter-skinned individuals form less protective pigment and are therefore more susceptible to sunburn, premature aging of the skin, and skin cancer after prolonged sun exposure. Red-heads are at particular risk, since they not only have the least pigment, but also their pheomelanin is far less protective than the melanin found in other skin types.

More and smarter cells

The epidermis contains two other very important specialized kinds of cells. The first line of defence of the body against foreign substances are the *Langerhans cells*, which are the "skin corps" of the body's immune system. They capture surface irritants to present them to the immune cells in the blood of the dermis below. It is these Langerhans cells that are responsible for skin allergies such as poison ivy, but in producing uncomfortable, itching blisters and rashes they protect our bodies from more serious consequences.

Merkel cells are special nerve cells that are most abundant in the fingertips, the lips, the gums, the palate, and the outer sheath of the hair follicle. Their interaction with nerves is responsible for our exquisite sensitivity, which hopefully gives us more pleasure than pain!

The dermis

The inner layer of your skin – the dermis – is on one hand tough, supporting the epidermis and resisting any tears, and on the other hand mobile, capable of extending and relaxing. It is

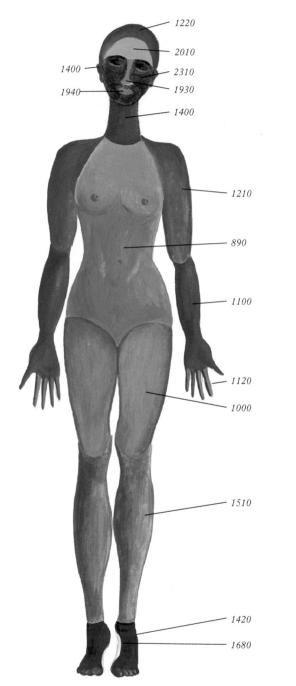

1220

2010

1400

2310

1940

1930

1400

1210

890

1100

1120

1000

1510

1420

1680

Skin pigmentation is not evenly distributed over your body – this chart shows the number of melanocytes per square millimetre.
Adapted from: Fitzpatrick T.B., Szabó G., "The melonocyte: cytology and cytochemistry", *Journal of Investigative Dermatology* 32, 197–209, 1959

thickest on the back of your body (about ³⁄₁₆ in or 4mm), and thinnest (surprisingly) on the palms of your hands (about ½in or 1mm). Your dermis is made up of three kinds of tissue: collagen, elastin, and ground substance.

Collagen

Collagen is the structural support of the dermis, making up 70 percent of its weight. In the upper or papillary dermis, collagen forms a loose network of relatively thin fibers that are parallel to the wavy ridges of the overlying epidermis. In the deeper or reticular dermis, the collagen fibres are thicker and the network of interconnecting fibres is denser and lies parallel to the skin. (See Chapter 10 to learn about collagen implants.)

Elastic fibres

Investigating further, interwoven between the strands of collagen are *elastic fibres* (which make the dermis pliable) and *reticulum fibres* (which add support), each made of specific proteins. It is the elastic fibres that allow our skin to stretch. Skin elasticity is what permits our skin to spring back to normal after weight gain, and what permits us to smile and make facial expressions.

Ground substance

All of the above structural fibres are embedded in the gel-like ground substance made of large molecules composed of proteins that are linked to sugars – *mucopolysaccharides*. Although these mucopolysaccharides comprise only 0.1 to 0.3 percent of the skin weight, each molecule can absorb a volume of water equal to as much as 1,000 times its volume!

These mucopolysaccharides not only serve as a support for the other components of the dermis and the subcutaneous tissue, but they are also like a sponge which plays a unique, key role in the salt and water balance of our body. When women retain water during phases of their menstrual cycle, or if your legs swell after sitting for a long time (especially on plane trips), the extra moisture is largely bound to these mucopolysaccharides, which often give the sensation of tight skin.

Mucopolysaccharides surround all of the dermal cells, including those that make collagen and elastin. Just as people's ways of behavior change depending on their surroundings, so do these cells modify their action on collagen and elastic tissue and change their ways of growing and developing depending on the makeup of the surrounding mucopolysaccharides. This recently discovered fact is at the centre of considerable research at present on ways to control or influence cell growth and may also prove of interest for skincare products.

Still more cells

Continuing our guided tour of the dermis, there is a variety of free cells, most prominently *fibroblasts,* which are scattered throughout the dermis, ready to fabricate (or "synthesize") collagen and elastin when needed. If the skin is cut, the fibroblasts whip into action to rebuild the damage. In a healing wound, many activated fibroblasts are seen at the injury sight, rapidly manufacturing new, fine fibrillar collagen. If the fibroblasts work overtime, an enlarged, hard scar can form, known as a "hypertrophic" scar or "keloid". These can be medically treated.

There are also some granular *mast cells* which reside near the blood vessels. When a foreign irritant appears, the mast cells shoot out granules which are like bullets full of enzymes that kill the intruder. More mast cells keep appearing on the scene until the irritant is literally liquidated. You will feel an itchy bump or hives on your skin as a result of this battle.

The piping system

Networks of nerves, blood vessels, and lymphatics (the drainage system) course through the dermis, all arising from and leading back to the larger nerves and vessels of the deeper, subcutaneous fat layer. The branching of these networks looks like a candelabra, with progressively thinner nerves and vessels reaching to the top layer of the dermis.

Each square inch of skin has more than 15ft (4.5m) of blood vessels, providing oxygen and other nutrients to the body, and removing carbon dioxide and other metabolic waste from the body. The pinker the area of skin, the more blood vessels there are: the lips and gums are particularly "vascular". Blood vessels expand with heat to cool the body by bringing more blood to the cooler surface; they also expand with nervousness and can cause that embarrassing blush. In the cold, the dermal blood vessels constrict to preserve body heat. This constriction is what can lead to frostbite in the fingertips, nose or ears.

The nerve system

Running alongside the blood vessels in the dermis are sensory nerves that convey sensations, and motor nerves that act on blood vessels, glands, and the tiny muscles that make each of our hairs stand on end with shivering. Specific sensory nerves have very delicate endings in the upper dermis, each of which detects one particular sensation, such as itching, pain or temperature. Also in the dermis are special receptor cells that were encountered in the epidermis. These are the *Merkel cells*, and receptor bodies (*Meissner* and *Pacinian corpuscles)* which recognize the size and shape of objects touched.

The skin gets pretty crowded: for instance, on one square inch of the dermis on your cheek there are approximately 30 nerves, 15 sensory receptors for cold, 80 receptors for heat, and 1,300 receptors for pain. And there are even more than this on the most sensitive areas of your body, such as the fingertips, lips and genitals. There's a lot more going on in your skin than you ever realized!

The glands are here

Also embedded in the dermis are three types of secretory glands, each of which is the source of some conditions with which you are, unfortunately, all too familiar. The *sebaceous* glands cause the oiliness of your face and hair, and can also help bring about those unwelcome pimples and blackheads. The *eccrine* glands generate sweat in reaction to heat, exercise, fever, and stress. The *apocrine* glands produce those body odors that we prefer to camouflage.

The sebaceous and apocrine glands secrete into our hair follicles, while the eccrine glands

have their own tiny openings onto the skin's surface. There is a tendency to worry not only about the secretions themselves, but also about the appearance of the openings – the pores. Especially on our faces, pores can appear prominent and unattractive. The size of our pores is largely hereditary, though with proper treatment their appearance can be reduced, as you will learn in Chapter 8.

The sebaceous glands have the important function of providing a protective covering of slightly acidic, natural oil which prevents excessive evaporation of water from the skin surface. The largest number and greatest size of sebaceous glands are on the face and scalp, followed by the back and chest. There are no hairs or sebaceous glands on the palms of our hands and the soles of our feet, partially explaining why these areas can suffer from very dry, cracked skin!

Importantly, the sebaceous glands are very sensitive to hormones, especially to the male hormones which increase the glands' size and the secretion of oil (*sebum*).

This is why males are more susceptible to acne, particularly in puberty! In contrast, the female hormone estrogen decreases the size of the gland and the production of oily sebum, while progesterone (especially when taken in medication such as an oral contraceptive) can increase sebaceous gland size. In men, oily secretion falls only slightly with age, whereas in women it decreases significantly after the age of 50.

There are two to four million eccrine sweat glands distributed over your entire body surface, with a larger number concentrated on the palms, soles and forehead. A person can perspire as much as 10 litres (over 2½ gal) each day. The main function of sweat is to cool the body down when it overheats from hot weather, exercise or fever. The duct leading to the sweat glands conserves salt, so sweat is mainly water; toxic heavy metals and organic compounds are also actively expelled. Interestingly, eccrine sweat does not contribute to body odor.

There's just one more interesting gland to take note of – the apocrine sweat gland, the exact function of which in humans is not fully understood. In other mammals, the odor of the apocrine (secretion) attracts a mate, acts as an identification signal to friends and enemies, and also marks territorial boundaries. The apocrine glands are found under the arm, in the genital and perianal areas, and around the belly button and nipples. After puberty, they secrete a milky, viscous fluid in response to: stress, surprise, fear or during intercourse. Although this secretion is odorless when first released, the skin surface bacteria rapidly feed on the apocrine fats to produce a pungent, unpleasant body odor.

The source of hair

Hair follicles are distributed over the entire body except for the palms and soles. Some follicles produce the thick, "terminal" hairs of the scalp, eyebrows, eyelashes, pubic areas, and of men's beards and body hair. Most hair follicles, however, grow tiny, barely perceptible vellus hairs. The hair is actually a long strand of overlapping layers of the protein keratin, which is very similar to the surface of your outer skin layer. Contrary to what you might think, the hair itself is not living; it is made up of dead tissue in the same way as our nails.

Hair is formed in the bulbous follicle at the base of the hair shaft deep in the dermis. In contrast to the well-marked pattern of molting that occurs in many animal species, hair growth on the human scalp is a kind of mosaic of follicular activity, with alternating periods of growth (*anagen*) and rest (*telogen*) separated by a transitional (*catogen*) phase.

Scalp hair grows about 0.3 mm each day, or about 4 inches (11cm) per year. To shed 50 to 100 hairs a day is considered normal. When hair is shed, it is replaced by new hair formed in the same follicle located just below the skin surface. New hair growth can be initiated by plucking the hair from a resting follicle or by wounding. Certain hormones, such as estrogen, progesterone, testosterone, and the thyroid hormone, also influence hair growth (and, regrettably, hair loss).

Your hair color is determined by the number and type of melanosomes that migrate into your hair bulbs.

How your skin ages

You've now learned a little about the composition, structure and function of your skin. Now it is time to look at how your skin is affected over the years.

Fortunately and unfortunately, our bodies are pre-programmed to age. Fortunately because, as we grow, we mature and become wiser and more self-sufficient. It is certainly not desirable to remain as five-year-olds throughout life, although it would be pleasant to spend a few worry-free days each month as a child! As to unfortunately, everyone understands the consequences of aging all too well, although we should keep in mind Maurice Chevalier's observation: "I prefer old age to the alternative."

As people age, it takes both knowledge and a sustained, daily skin program to maintain the good health and appearance that we took for granted for so many years. The bad news is that we will develop wrinkles and age spots on our skin, and our hair will become thinner and turn gray. The good news is that this book will share with you the major advances of medical science in understanding how to prevent or slow down many of the unattractive aspects of aging, especially skin aging.

Natural aging

There are two kinds of skin aging. The first is the inevitable, natural, biologic aging programmed into our cells, the so-called "intrinsic aging". The precise path along which we age varies for each of us and is determined by our genetics – i.e. how we "choose" our parents. The skin of different races and of different individuals within one race, indeed even within one family, shows their true age to varying degrees. In general, darker skins show age less than lighter skins.

By observing your parents, you will have a good idea of how your skin will age. If you follow my skincare program, you should easily be able to slow down this natural intrinsic aging.

The damage we do

The second kind of aging of the skin is "extrinsic aging", an aging over which we have more control. Extrinsic aging is the acceleration of intrinsic aging caused by various environmental conditions, primarily exposure to the UV sun rays. Extrinsic skin damage can be blamed on the accumulation of external events that are bad for your skin, rather than on normal wear and tear or passing time. As you will learn in Chapter 4, sun exposure is responsible for so-called photoaging of the skin and causes 90 percent of the damage.

If you wish to observe first-hand the two very distinct kinds of skin aging, just look at the difference between the skin on the inside of your arm near the armpit, and the skin on the top of your hand. Anyone over 30 will notice that his or her skin on the inner arm is supple and smooth, almost like a baby's skin, quite different from that on the sun-exposed hand. These noticeable differences are due to the different cellular and molecular processes of the two types of aging.

As shown in Table 1, intrinsic aging is characterized by "less" and extrinsic aging by "more". Where skin ages normally it just seems to wind down, whereas in extrinsically aged skin all the processes accelerate, to protect us.

What this aging means

With intrinsic biological aging, the skin's outer layer is thinned (over time by about 20 percent). The surface of the skin remains smooth. The border between the epidermis and the dermis becomes flattened, making the skin less resistant to friction (you get more blisters in snug shoes!). In contrast, extrinsic photoaging causes a thickening of the outer skin layer, with up to 50 percent more cells being accumulated onto the skin's surface, making it feel rough and dry. Think of the grainy, thickened skin on the backs of the hands of a gardener, for example. With photoaging, accumulation of pigment in the basal cells is more markedly irregular than in intrinsic aging, causing the so-called "liver spots" or "age spots" (medically called *solar lentigos*), the unattractive dark spots especially prevalent on the hands, arms, face and chest.

Even greater differences between intrinsic and extrinsic aging are seen in the skin's inner layer,

the dermis. The most noticeable distinction is that in photoaged skin, the elastic fibres are markedly increased and thickened. This is not seen in normal, protected skin, in which elastic fibres may increase slightly in quantity and thickness but maintain the normal candelabra-like pattern of fibres.

This so-called *solar-elastosis* effect is readily observed on the thick, leathery skin on the neck of a fisherman: deep wrinkles are fixed and prominent, and the skin is not very pliable. At the same time, the amount of mature collagen in photoaged skin decreases and the dermis is filled with degenerated elastic fibres and increased amounts of the gel-like substance – the

Table 1: Comparison of Skin Changes with Natural Aging and Sun Damage

What You See			What Is Seen in a Microscope		
	Sun Damage *(Extrinsic)*	Natural Aging *(Intrinsic)*		Sun Damage *(Extrinsic)*	Natural Aging *(Intrinsic)*
Skin Surface	Wrinkles, coarse and fine	Wrinkles, fine			
			Epidermis	Thickened	Thinned
Texture	Rough	Smooth	Stratum corneum	Very thickened	Not thickened
Pigmentation	Mottled dark spots "liver spots"	Pale	Basal pigment cells	Increased and clumped	Not increased or clumped
			Dermis		
Skin thickness	Leathery, thick	Smooth, thin	Elastic fibres	Markedly increased clumped, - disoriented	Minimally decreased, not clumped Not disorientated
			MPS's*-	Increased	Decreased
			Fibroblasts	Active	Inactive
Skin	Sallow	Pale			
	Mottled redness Tetangectasia (tiny blood vessels)	Evenly pink	Blood vessels	Dilated and tortuous	Decreased, Not dilated
			Inflammation	Frequently	None
Pores	Dilated with blackheads and whiteheads	Not dilated	Hair follicles	Dilated, filled with horny debris	Atrophy
			Sebaceous glands	Enlarged	Atrophy
Growths	Seborrheic keratoses Actinic keratoses Carcinoma (basal and squamous) Melanoma	Senile angiomas			

*MPS's = mucopolysaccharides

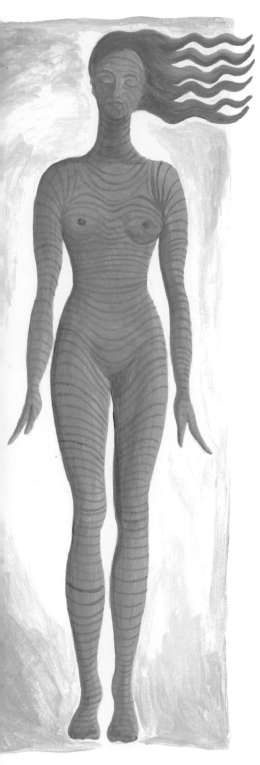

mucopolysaccharide – that surrounds these fibres. The composition of this gel is different from youthful skin. With normal, biologic aging, these mucopolysaccharides decrease.

Another major difference in photoaged skin is the presence of many cells. Fibroblasts, white blood cells and mast cells abound, all working overtime to repair the extrinsic damage they encountered. As mentioned, the presence of all of these cells means that photoaged skin is chronically red and inflamed. In contrast, with natural aging there are fewer cells because all this activity has slowed down.

Blood circulation in the skin also suffers from both natural aging and sun exposure. In protected aged skin, the number of small blood vessels declines, but those remaining are not unnaturally expanded and are normal. With photoaging, these micro-blood vessels become misshapen. With normal aging, the decline in the efficiency of the skin's "drainage system" (its "lymphatics") is just moderate, whereas with photodamage, this loss is so marked that the lymphatics are practically absent.

Hair follicles normally degenerate with age, as do sebaceous glands. In contrast, after photodamage through sun exposure, follicles expand and fill with debris from the sun-thickened layer of outer skin. This in turn makes the sebaceous glands become greatly enlarged, leading to more oily secretion and unsightly blackheads.

Certain marks or growths become more visible with aging. The dominant marking normally associated with age is a little red dot or soft, red raised papule, the so-called *senile angioma*, occurring most frequently on the trunk of the body. Rarely do other growths occur in sun-protected skin. In contrast, as you will learn in Chapter 6, various unsightly growths can appear on the skin almost exclusively in areas exposed to UV light, including wart-like growths (seborrheic keratoses), rough spots (*actinic keratoses*), and skin cancers.

Wrinkles and aging

Even young children have wrinkles! All skin has folds corresponding to the way the skin envelops and moves with the body, as shown in the illustration on this page and opposite. To minimize the appearance of scars, when surgeons make incisions in the skin they follow the direction of these so-called *Langer's lines* whenever possible.

When you look closely at your skin, you can see tiny furrows that intersect in complex ways, creating delicate skin-surface patterns which vary with age and differ from one part of the body to another. In unexposed areas of young people's skin, these patterns are orderly and regular. With intrinsic aging, the furrows become shallower and the pattern becomes more irregular in shape. Where skin has been exposed to the sun, there is a loss of skin-surface pattern with age.

With both intrinsic and extrinsic aging, the amount of fat under the skin steadily decreases. The degree of fat absorption varies in different parts of the body. The combination of decreased thickness of the dermis, decreased resilience of the skin, and the loss of subcutaneous fat makes sagging skin and jowl-like wrinkles become more apparent.

We all shrink from the moment we stop growing. This contraction of bone usually accelerates in our late 50s or early 60s. Particularly prominent is some contraction of our facial structure causing sagging jowls and wrinkles; this is further accentuated by the later loss of teeth. Our skin can then begin to fold away from the underlying muscle and bone, and gravity pulls that excessive, non-resilient skin down.

In Chapter 9 you will learn how some wrinkles can be prevented, or at least the onset can be retarded, by changing some personal skincare habits and by using certain treatments at home. Chapter 10 describes how a dermatologist or plastic surgeon can do even more to help keep you looking young.

Skin science

By now you will have learned that the skin is a marvellous and complex machine. As with any good machine, only regular care and maintenance can assure good service and give the very best appearance. In this book, I am happy to share with you some secrets and some easy and effective measures for keeping your skin looking excellent and as young as possible. This is a program that not only works but is great for your health as well!

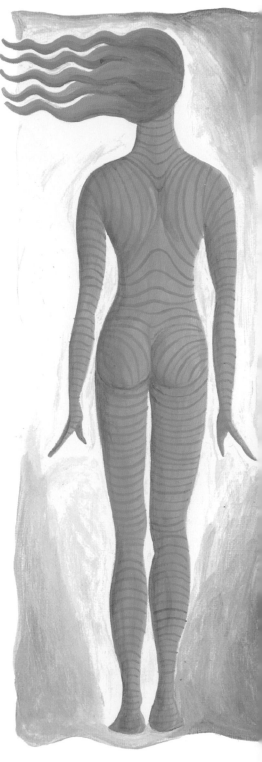

The skin surface folds along natural lines.
To minimize scars, surgeons cut along these lines whenever possible.
Adapted from: Kraisel C.J., "The selection of appropriate lines for elective incisions",
Plastic and Reconstructive Surgery 8: 1–28, 1951

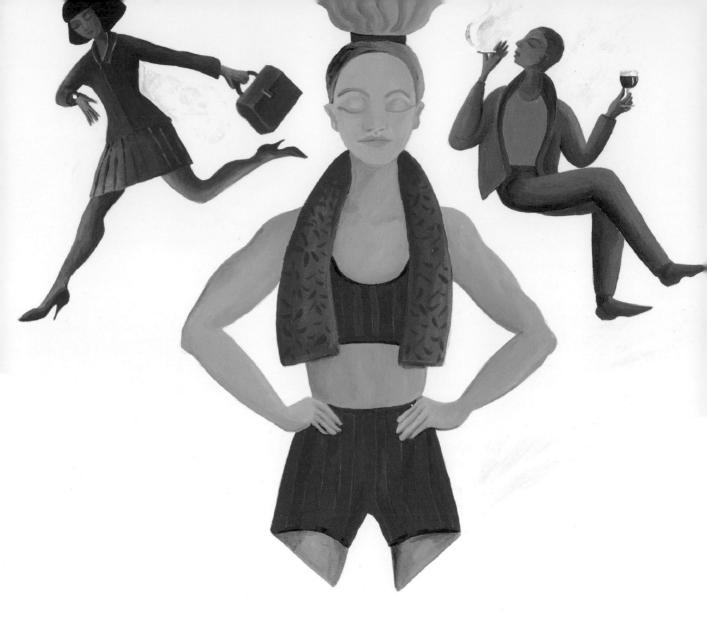

A Personal Skin Analysis

We are all individuals, with a skin like no one else's! Although most of our
physical attributes are largely predetermined by our parents, we do not
need to be a slave to our biological makeup. Today more than ever, we all
understand how our lifestyle may influence our overall health, including
our skin, during each phase of our lives. Recent scientific research about
cosmetics and skincare has given us products and techniques to
prevent and improve almost all skin problems.

On the following pages are three questionnaires that will help you analyze your skin in a different way from before. The mistake that everyone can make in determining their skin type is not taking enough time to do it properly and rigorously. These questions will help you think about all parts of your skin, including your body as well as your face. You will realize how your overall health, past and present, can influence your skin. You will think in detail about your present lifestyle and your diet. If you have a particular problem, you may even realize its cause by just answering these questions. And although no test can predict definitively how any one individual will age, some questions will highlight the major factors influencing the appearance of aging.

These questions may suggest subtle changes you can make in your habits or your environment – both now and in future years – which can markedly improve your skin in ways that you may not hitherto have considered.

Answering all these questions without self-criticism will help you identify your problem areas. It will make you notice ways in which your lifestyle can influence your skin in ways that you did not previously imagine.

What kind of skin do you have?

1   How old are you? _____

Everyone's skin changes with different phases in life, influenced especially by hormones, diet, environment and lifestyle.

2   How would you characterize your race and that of your parents?

	Self	Mother	Father		Self	Mother	Father
Black	___	___	___	Indian (American)	___	___	___
Caucasian	___	___	___	Indian (India)	___	___	___
Hispanic	___	___	___	Filipino	___	___	___
Mediterranean	___	___	___	Oriental	___	___	___

Every race has its advantages and disadvantages with respect to the skin. The Great Skin for Life skincare program will teach you how to "accentuate the positive", as Johnny Mercer's song advises.

3   What are the colors of your skin and eyes?

Skin:	White (porcelain)___	White (olive) ___	Black (medium) ___	Yellow ___
	White (freckled) ___	Black (light) ___	Black (dark) ___	Red ___
Eyes:	Brown ___	Blue ___	Green ___	Hazel ___

What is the natural color of your hair?

Black ___   Blonde ___   Brown ___   Chestnut ___   Red ___   Gray ___

In general, the lighter your skin, eyes, and hair, the more sensitive your skin. Red-heads and blondes with freckles are the most sensitive, especially to the sun.

4   How would your describe your sensitivity to the sun?

I   Always burns, never tans
II   Always burns, then slightly tans
III   Sometimes burns, always tans
IV   Never burns, always tans
V   Heavily pigmented: never burns
VI   Black: never burns

Individuals with type I and type II skin have light skin color, blue eyes, and often red hair and sometimes freckling. Some people with dark brown hair and blue or green eyes can have type I and type II reactions to the sun. Everyone should cover up, especially if you ever burn! (Modified from Committee on Impacts of Stratospheric Change: Halocarbons: Environmental Effects of Cholofluoromethane Release. Washington DC National Academy of Sciences, 1976.)

5 Have you ever had X-ray or Grenz treatments to your skin?
yes/no   age ____ number of treatments ____

Although X-ray treatments are occasionally used to treat skin diseases, the skin can react even years later. Be sure to tell your dermatologist about all such previous treatments.

6. Has your skin changed recently? yes/no   If so, how?

	Location		Location		Location
Oiliness	_____	Acne	_____	Sensitivity to sun	_____
Dryness	_____	Hives	_____	Sensitivity to cosmetics	_____
Rough, scaly patches	_____	Redness/Flushing	_____	Excess hair	_____
Dandruff	_____	New blood vessels	_____	New moles	_____
Itch	_____	Fungal infection	_____	Skin cancer	_____

If your skin has changed you may learn why as you read the questions below pertaining to your lifestyle.

7 Have you or anyone in your immediate family had any of the following skin problems? At what age did you or your relative have this problem? Was it treated by a dermatologist?

	You	Family	Treatment		You	Family	Treatment
Acne	__	__	_____	Flushing	__	__	_____
Dry skin	__	__	_____	Excessive perspiration	__	__	_____
Seborrhea or dandruff	__	__	_____	Body odor	__	__	_____
Atopic dermatitis/eczema	__	__	_____	Alopecia (hair loss)	__	__	_____
Contact dermatitis	__	__	_____	Hirsutism (excess hair)	__	__	_____
Bacterial infections	__	__	_____	Excessive bleeding when cut	__	__	_____
Fungal Infections	__	__	_____	Excessive or frequent bruising	__	__	_____
Herpes (zoster or simplex)	__	__	_____	Difficulty with wound healing	__	__	_____
Hives	__	__	_____	Overgrown scars or keloids	__	__	_____
Rashes	__	__	_____	New moles	__	__	_____
Psoriasis	__	__	_____	Skin cancer	__	__	_____

All of these conditions definitely require a visit to a dermatologist! Some of these skin problems could indicate systemic conditions which should be investigated, others can be easily treated. Remember, the sooner you see the doctor, the sooner your skin will improve!

8 Medical History: have you ever had any of the following?

	Yes/No	Age		Yes/No	Age
Anaphylaxis*	__	__	Blood or lymph gland disorder	__	__
Allergies (to food, drugs, plants)	__	__	Phlebitis	__	__
Neurological disorder	__	__	Arthritis, joint problems or bone disease	__	__
Fainting	__	__	Cancer	__	__
Convulsions	__	__	Frequent infections	__	__
Eye disease	__	__	Diabetes	__	__
Heart disease	__	__	Thyroid disorder	__	__
Hypertension	__	__	Ovarian or testicular disorder	__	__
Hay fever, asthma	__	__	Irregular, very painful, or excessive menstrual periods	__	__
Lung disease	__	__	Venereal disease	__	__
Liver or gall bladder disease	__	__	Adrenal disease	__	__
Ulcers, gastrointestinal disease	__	__	Other hormonal disorder	__	__
Urinary or bladder problems	__	__	Auto-immune disease**	__	__
Kidney disease	__	__	Emotional or psychiatric problems	__	__

*   swelling, difficulty breathing or passing out after an insect bite of ingestion of food or medication
**   lupus erythematosus, dermatomyositis, poylmositis, Hashimoto's thyroiditis, scleroderma, ulcerative colitis, Crohn's disease, Sjogren's syndrome, Reiter's syndrome, mixed connective tissue

All of these medical problems can directly affect your skin. Usually treatment of the underlying condition cures any skin involvement.

How does your lifestyle affect your skin?

1 Do you work primarily indoors?   yes/no

When indoors, are you usually in a sealed building, or is there always fresh air? _____

Statistics show that the average urban worker spends 90 prcent of his or her time indoors in tightly sealed buildings where air is dry and recirculated , which is certainly not good for the skin!

2 Do you work with irritating chemicals such as cleaning solutions, volatile solvents, or paints?   yes/no

Do you handle many papers — either newsprint or copy-machine copies?   yes/no

Chemicals that you touch either directly or on paper and newspapers are quite irritating to your skin, especially if those irritants are inadvertently rubbed onto your face by your hands.

3 Did you ever get a rash or other irritation?   yes/no

after new curtains or carpets were installed? _____
after a room was painted or a floor was polished? _____

If you answered "yes" to any of these questions, you may be sensitive to formaldehyde or other volatile solvents.

4 Did you ever get a rash   yes/no   yes/no

under earrings?	_____	under a watch?	_____
under a bracelet?	_____	under a hat?	_____
under a ring?	_____	on your soles when wearing no socks?	_____
under a necklace?	_____	under the elastic of your underwear?	_____

If you answered "yes", you might be allergic either to nickel or to a component of leather or elastic or synthetic material.

5 Have you ever had a rash after touching poison ivy or sumac? or other plants? yes/no

Do you have allergies to pollen? yes/no   ragweed? yes/no   other plants yes/no

Do you garden or work with plants? yes/no   Take long walks in wooded areas? yes/no

We are all aware of any severe allergies we may have to certain plants, but we are less aware of cross-reactions between these plants and other commonly used substances. For instance, anyone allergic to ragweed might be sensitive to chamomile or arnica; individuals allergic to poison ivy or sumac may react to cashew nuts or oil.

6 Do you exercise regularly? yes/no   What exercise do you do?

	hours each week		hours each week		hours each week
Bicycle riding	_____	Swimming	_____	Golf	_____
Calisthenics	_____	Yoga	_____	Tennis	_____
Walking	_____	Running	_____	Other	_____

Exercise is great for your body and for your skin, but it can have adverse effects from excessive sweating, blistering, or be irritated from chlorinated or salt water. You will learn how to recognize and solve these problems in Chapter 8.

7 Do you regularly use cosmetics? Have you ever had an irritation or rash after using them?

	use	irritation		use	irritation		use	irritation
Foundation makeup	_	_____	Day creams	_	_____	Deodorant or antiperspirant	_	_____
Eye shadow	_	_____	Night creams	_	_____	Body powders	_	_____
Mascara	_	_____	Body lotions	_	_____	Perfumes	_	_____
Blush	_	_____	Soaps or cleansers	_	_____	Shampoos	_	_____
Powder	_	_____	Cleansing creams	_	_____	Hair conditioners	_	_____
Other makeup	_	_____	Masques	_	_____	Hair gels/ spray	_	_____

Any cosmetic or perfume or skincare product, even if it is labeled "oil free" or "hypoallergenic" might cause acne or a rash or photosensitivity in certain individuals. If you do have any new rash or irritation, think first about what products you might have applied!

8 Do you take frequent steam baths? yes/no Do you sit in jacuzzis or hot baths? yes/no

Although this heat feels good and gives your skin a rosy glow, with time it can cause extra blood vessels to form on your face and/or legs. If you have the type of skin that flushes, you should avoid this excessive heat.

9 How many hours do you sleep each night? _____   How variable is this? _____

Do you sleep on your side or back or stomach, or do you toss and turn? _____

Do you sleep with your head elevated? _____   How many pillows do you use? _____

How often do you feel fatigued? *Every day* ___ *Several times each week* ___ *Never* ___

Do you take naps? _____   Do you nap in bed or elsewhere? _____

Most of us sleep for at least one-fourth to one-third of our lives, and sometimes even more. Our sleeping position affects how rested and invigorated we feel upon awakening. You will learn how to make your resting sleep a real "beauty sleep".

How does your diet affect your skin?

1 Do you take any of these vitamins?

	Amount/day	# years		Amount/day	# years		Amount/day	# years
Vitamin A	____	____	Vitamin E	____	____	Zinc	____	____
Vitamin B	____	____	Beta-carotene	____	____	Multivitamins	____	____
Vitamin C	____	____	Selenium	____	____	Other	____	____

All of these vitamins can be good for your skin, as you will learn in Chapter 8.

2 Do you habitually drink alcohol or caffeinated beverages? yes/no

Alcohol - type	____	Caffeine - coffee	____ cups/day
amount/day	____	tea	____ cups/day
amount/week	____	soft drinks	____ cups/day

Alcohol and caffeine can cause flushing or redness of the face, especially if taken excessively.

3. Do you regularly take   aspirin? yes/no,   indomethacin? yes/no,
codeine? yes/no,   steroids? yes/no

Aspirin and codeine can increase a tendency to get hives; indomethacin and steroids decrease the incidence of hives and other allergies. However, steroids can cause acne, bleeding ulcers, decreased immunity to infections, abnormalities in blood sugar, as well as other serious medical problems. They should be taken only very carefully under a doctor's close supervision.

4 Do you get acne or hives after eating any of these foods?

	acne	hives		acne	hives		acne	hives
cheese*	___	___	milk*	___	___	shellfish	___	___
citrus fruits	___	___	nuts*	___	___	strawberries	___	___
chocolate*	___	___	pork	___	___	tomatoes	___	___
corn	___	___	seasonings	___	___	wheat	___	___
eggs	___	___	ice cream*	___	___	yogurt*	___	___

*The foods labelled with * frequently cause acne and/or hives; the others are often the culprits in causing hives. Blue cheese and Roquefort cheese are particular offenders, not only because they are very rich but also because they contain penicillin, a common allergen.*

How will your skin age?

1   Where did you live until you were 18 years old? _____

Was your skin exposed to the sun and/or extreme dryness or cold?   yes/no

Did you travel to hot, sunny climates, particularly in the winter? yes/no How often?_____

Especially your early environment influences your skin decades later.

2   Did you ever sunbathe or use a tanning salon?   yes/no

Did you ever get a blistering sunburn?   yes/no   How many times? _____

Do you use a high SPF sunscreen whenever you are exposed to the sun? yes/no

All sun prematurely ages your skin! One blistering sunburn as a child doubles the probability of skin cancer! It is never too late to protect yourself against this needless premature aging and damage to your skin.

3   Do you ride in a car more than three hours each week? yes/no

Are you more frequently the driver or the passenger? _____

You can be inadvertently exposed to the sun as you ride in cars. Often this is obvious because the skin of the hands, arms and face appears older on the side of sun exposure. Whether you drive or ride, don't forget that sunscreen – especially one that protects against UVA, which is not blocked by glass as is UVB.

4   Is your complexion freckled, light, olive, yellow or dark? _____

Is your skin oily or dry? _____

In general, the darker your skin and the less dry, the better your skin will age.

5   Did your mother and/or father appear to age faster than their peers? yes/no

Did they spend a lot of time in the sun, unprotected by sunscreen?   yes/no

If your parents look younger than their peers, you are lucky! You may have inherited those good genes. If they appear older, it could be partially because they did not know, as you do, the importance of sun protection. Fortunately, you can benefit from their example.

6   Does your weight frequently fluctuate by more than ten pounds? yes/no

Do you habitually binge, then diet? yes/no

Repeatedly losing and regaining weight can lead to stretch marks and lax, sagging skin. Avoiding yo-yo dieting saves your face as well as your body.

7   Do you drink alcohol with meals? yes/no Between meals? yes/no

What alcoholic beverages do you drink?_____ How much each week?_____

Excess alcohol causes rosacea, flushing, and permanent small blood vessels. And no one needs all those extra calories!

8   Do you smoke? yes/no How many cigarettes do you smoke each day? _____

What type of cigarettes? _____ Do you live or work with someone who smokes? yes/no

All smoking or exposure to someone else's cigarette smoke prematurely ages your skin! If the damage to your lungs is not enough to influence you to stop smoking, the adverse effects on your skin should!

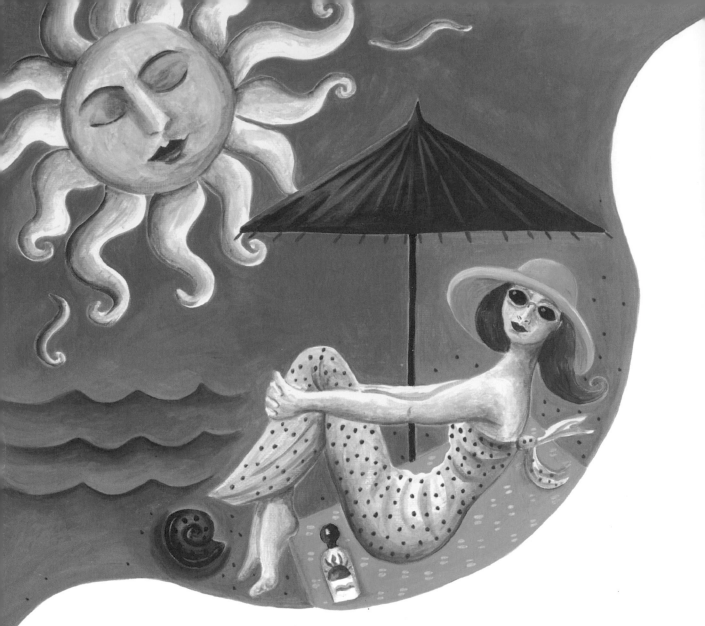

Sun Safety

On sunny days most of us are filled with a sense of joy and wellbeing. Our cares seem to melt away in a sea of brightness. In the far north, when short winter days bring little sun, people suffer from increased depression. Let's admit it: sunshine feels good and makes us feel good. The sun's warming rays are responsible for life on earth evolving as it has. In fact without the sun's heat people wouldn't exist. But the sun is a fickle friend, which can do considerable damage if your are not on your guard. The trick is to learn to enjoy the sun without letting it harm you.

Plants need the sun for growth, but do we? In truth, someone eating a severely vitamin-deficient diet would require about 20 minutes of sun exposure each day for their skin to synthesize vitamin D. With the exception of those in very underdeveloped countries and people who "survive" on junk food, everyone gets sufficient vitamin D from their normal diet. Physiologically, therefore, we do not need the sun.

Virtually all the other effects of exposure to the sun are damaging, especially to our skin and eyes. That is why simple rules of sun safety should be a vital part of everyone's daily fitness routine. Sun safety is as important as exercise and diet to maintain both good health and an attractive appearance.

The tanning myth

When and why did tanning become popular? In the last century, a tan was definitely not considered to be "chic": only laborers, farmers, and fishermen who worked long hours outdoors had tans. Women of the "upper classes" took particular pride in their porcelain-white, unspotted skins, protecting themselves from the sun with parasols, gloves, and large hats. Female beauty was measured by the translucence and smoothness of the skin.

The attitude towards tanning began to change as late as the 1920s, when Coco Chanel first caused a sensation in Paris and around the world by showing her haute couture clothing on tanned models.

A golden tan soon became a fashionable symbol of travel and of a luxurious life of leisurely vacations in the sun. As the notion of the ideal evolved and the active outdoor lifestyle became preferred, tanned skin has more recently been viewed as an emblem of healthy athletic fitness and prowess.

Medical science has now proved beyond doubt that the sun not only noticeably accelerates the visible aging of skin, but that it also causes distinct, irreversible skin damage and also disease. Despite broad media coverage making the public aware of these dangers, tanning lotions still sell well and, unfortunately, tanning salons still make a good living.

A recent survey by an American women's magazine showed that although over 85 percent of Americans are aware that the radiation from the sun's rays is unhealthy, only about half of them actually take precautions to protect themselves from its effects. Another survey by the newspaper *USA Today* found that 80 percent of people on vacation chose their destination primarily to get maximum sun exposure!

Gradually styles are changing, albeit at a slow pace. Fashion models today are shown without tans, unlike those who were pictured ten years or so ago. Inspired by our newly acquired knowledge, our concept of "beauty" is slowly returning to a much healthier balance.

Solar radiation – "the ultra-V three"

Sunlight is electromagnetic radiation, which is similar to X-rays but of lower energy. The sun's energy reaching the earth's surface can be broadly subdivided into 1) infrared (the lowest energy that can be felt as heat); 2) visible light; and 3) ultraviolet (the highest energy that affects

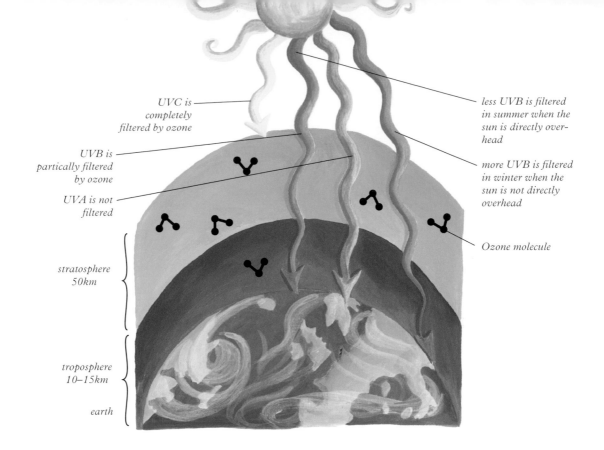

UVC is
completely
filtered by ozone

UVB is
partically filtered
by ozone

UVA is not
filtered

stratosphere
50km

troposphere
10–15km

earth

less UVB is filtered
in summer when the
sun is directly over-
head

more UVB is filtered
in winter when the
sun is not directly
overhead

Ozone molecule

the skin). The ultraviolet spectrum is, in turn, divided into three bands – the "ultra-V three" – each of which causes a different, specific, and most unwelcome effect.

UVC

The highest energy ultraviolet band, ultraviolet C (UVC), is potentially the most damaging to skin, but all of this ultraviolet C is screened by the ozone layer high in the earth's atmosphere. This radiation is very dangerous, in fact, UVC lamps are actually used in biological laboratories and operating rooms to disinfect and kill germs!

UVB

The mid-energy range is ultraviolet B (UVB). UVB energy causes the most serious damage to the skin because its wavelengths interact directly with the DNA of our genes. It is the UVB that is

most intense in the midday sun and in summer when the sun is closest to the earth. UVB radiation causes sunburn, wrinkles, unattractive dark spots, and also skin cancer.

UVA

Ultraviolet A (UVA) is the lowest energy range of ultraviolet radiation. Contrary to previous beliefs, UVA is far from harmless. Unlike UVB, which in temperate latitudes only significantly penetrates the atmosphere between 10am–4pm (with marked increases in summer months), levels of UVA are virtually constant throughout the day and throughout the year.

There is much more UVA than UVB reaching us at any one moment (by a factor ranging from 100- to 1000-fold, depending on time of day, season, and geographic location). UVA radiation even penetrates glass, so you are exposed when you stand near a window or travel in a car.

Although UVA may be the least damaging of the ultra-V three, it penetrates the skin more deeply than UVB, reaching right down to the dermis where it destroys collagen and elastic tissue and causes those dreaded wrinkles along with decreased elasticity and the appearance of aging. UVA is the cause of potentially serious photosensitizing reactions (see below). To make matters worse, UVA suppresses the skin's immune system, thereby increasing susceptibility to infections and possibly skin cancer.

The aggressive and intrusive combination of UVA and UVB radiation is out there, waiting to do damage to your skin and body, and in the longer term to threaten your health. This book will show you ways of enjoying outdoor pursuits while protecting yourself from the worst of the ill-effects posed by this menacing radiation.

Dangers of sun exposure

It is truly more dangerous now than even a few years ago to expose yourself to the sun! Scien-

tists have noted a substantial decrease in the ozone layer above the earth's atmosphere. This is the layer that acts as a protective filter to save us from the sun's harmful ultraviolet rays.

Measurements in the late fall, winter, and early spring of 1991 showed a reduction of 5 percent as opposed to the previous decade. Calibrations initially focused on the seasonal "hole" in the ozone layer, as tall as Mount Everest and as wide as the United States, which occurs over the Antarctic each September and October. Later studies by the US Environmental Program (USEP) reported that the earth's protective ozone layer has shrunk worldwide by about 4 percent in winter and 1 percent in summer.

Part of this ozone depletion may be due to the release into the atmosphere of chemical chloro-fluorocarbons from refrigerants and aerosol sprays (where they persist for over 90 years). Worldwide legislation is now severely limiting this modern hazard. A great part of the decrease in ozone may be as a result of natural cyclical variations in the earth's atmosphere, caused primarily

Table 1: The consequences of UVA and UVB exposure

UVA Radiation	UVB Radiation
CONSEQUENCES	
1 Sunburn, if excessive (as in tanning salons)	1 Sunburn
2 Suntan	2 Suntan
3 Premature aging: wrinkles, dark spots loss of elasticity	3 Premature aging: rough skin dark spots
4 Phototoxicity and photoallergy	4 Activation of viruses
5 Enhanced growth of: skin precancers skin cancers	5 Initiation of: skin precancers skin cancers
6 Decreased immunity of skin	

by the sun's gaseous emissions.

Whatever the causes, real or imagined, of the measurable decrease in the earth's ozone shield, the consequences to our skin are very real. The most dramatic effect is the marked increase in skin cancer. The number of skin cancers has *doubled* in each decade for the past 50 years. Also the number of deaths due to skin cancer have increased more than deaths due to any other cancer. One in six Americans will develop a skin cancer in his or her lifetime, and one in every three cancers diagnosed is skin cancer!

It is both encouraging, but also frustrating, that to a large extent this increase in skin cancer results from our voluntary behaviour and can thus easily be slowed and even reversed! Although there is depletion of the protective ozone layer and a consequent increase in the amount of UV radiation getting through to us, most of the increase in skin cancer actually results from our own changing lifestyles.

Everyone now has more leisure time to spend on outdoor activities both at home and away. People can be exposed to the sun in all seasons.

They can go skiing in winter (with extra reflection of sun from snow) and do outdoor sports such as tennis and golf in the spring and summer. Increased wealth and the accessibility of air travel allows us to move easily from northern regions to sunny climates for bursts of sun exposure, and today people are also more likely to take their children along.

In the course of just a two-week vacation in a sunny location, a northern European who works indoors doubles his or her annual dose of UVB radiation. To approximate to this doubling of UV exposure, were this same individual to forego the sun-filled vacation, the ozone layer would have to have been depleted by 50 percent! The good news is that only minor changes in our leisure habits can lead to major improvements in the health of our skin!

How dangerous is the sun?

There is no doubt that the sun does damage the skin. "If you tan now, you'll pay later!"

You will be surprised to learn about the many kinds of sun damage that you or your friends or family may suffer if you do not take the proper precautions. You were probably unaware of some of these hazards.

Sunburn

Although most people admit that they'd like a light suntan, nobody wants a *sunburn*. Nevertheless there are many people who love to spend hours at the beach, thinking that their sunburn is the first step towards a "glorious" tan. Many people have at one time shared this view. Nothing could be farther from the truth. The series of

Table 2

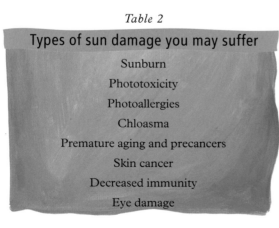

Types of sun damage you may suffer

Sunburn

Phototoxicity

Photoallergies

Chloasma

Premature aging and precancers

Skin cancer

Decreased immunity

Eye damage

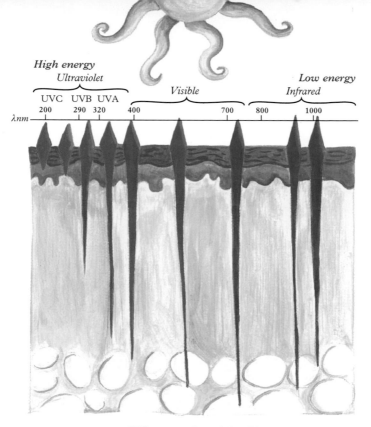

UV penetration of the skin
Shorter, high–energy UVC and UVB rays are absorbed
by the epidermis, longer UVA and visible rays penetrate
to the dermis and subcutaneous fat.

events that causes the sunburn in our skin, which results from too much sun exposure, is quite different from the mechanism of tanning. Sunburn is quite literally a "burn", just like a burn from hot water. Our surface blood vessels dilate (hence the redness), and inflammatory cells release the enzymes that fight the damage, causing blisters in the process.

As many of you have learned the hard way, the severe redness of a burn appears two to eight hours after our exposure to strong, usually midday, sun either during the summer or during a winter sun vacation or skiing. Blistering can occur after 12–24 hours of sun exposure. There is also redness that lasts up to a week, followed by severe peeling. Sometimes a person can experience *sunstroke,* with fever, chills and joint pain.

With sunburn, however, the worst is yet to come. Our skin cells "remember" the burn for ever, since in the healing process in which our DNA is cut and repaired, the repair may not be perfectly accomplished. Any minuscule error in the repair can reappear years later as a skin precancer or cancer.

If you accidentally fall asleep in the sun without putting on protection, or unexpectedly absorb reflected rays from water, snow or even concrete, there are several ways you can partially alleviate the sunburn. Adding oatmeal to a tepid bath or applying cool compresses may relieve and help to soothe the skin. Emollient creams give relief and help the dryness. Creams with menthol or phenol cool and reduce the pain to some extent.

Over-the-counter hydrocortisone preparations help to reduce the itching and burning. On the other hand, avoid lotions and sprays that contain anything ending in "-caine" anesthetics (especially benzocaine), since they can cause allergic reactions. In fact you should only use such preparations if you know you are not allergic.

Natural vitamin E (the *d-alpha-tocopheryl* acetate or succinate forms, but not the dl mixed tocopheryls) decreases the inflammation of sunburn. Taking 400 International Units (IU) (about one tablet) each day gives a sunscreen protection of about SPF 4 to your skin. If you are an adult exposed accidentally to excess sun and fear the onset of a sunburn, you should take 400 IU as soon as possible and every four hours thereafter for one or two days.

Alternatively, you can take one or two aspirins every four hours (if you have no problem with stomach ulcers or bruising) for one day to alleviate the inflammation of sunburn. Children over four years old could be given doses of vitamin E or aspirin proportional to their weight, but in all cases check the correct advisability and dosage with your doctor.

Phototoxicity

Phototoxicity is the unpleasant reaction that *all* people suffer when exposed to sunlight (primarily UVA) after having applied essences of particular plants or chemicals to the skin. This reaction can also occur after having eaten certain foods or taken certain medicines. There would be no adverse reaction if only a small amount of the offending substance was taken or applied and if

Table 3

Some Photosensitizing Medicines - A Partial List

(Specific Brand Names in Parentheses)

Antibacterial Soaps and Deodorants
   halogenatal salicylanilides

Antibacterial Agents
   sulfanilamide
   sulfacitamide
   sulfadiazine

Antibiotics
   demeclocycline
   doxycycline
   minocycline
   tetracycline
   tetracycline derivatives

Antidepressants
   amitriptyline (Elavil)
   desipramine (Norpramin)
   protriplyline (Vivactil)

Antidiabetic Medication
   tolbutamide (Orinase)

Antihistamines
   cyproheptadine (Periactin)
   diphenhydramine (Benadryl)

Antifungal Medication
   griseofuluin

Birth Control Pills
   estrogen

Cardiac Medicine
   quinidine

Diuretics
   chlorothiazide (Diuril)
   flurosemide (Lasix)
   triamterene (Dyazide)

Tranquillizers
   chlordiazepoxide (Librium)
   chlorpromazine (Thorazine)
   haloperidon (Haldol)
   thiothixene (Navane)

Urinary Antiseptic
   nalidoxic acid

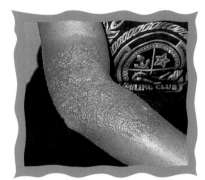

After taking an antibiotic and exposing her arm to sunlight, this woman suffered a severe photoallergy.
Science Photo Library, London

there was no exposure to the sun or a tanning bed.

A phototoxic response is usually immediate and can be most uncomfortable, with burning, redness, and often hives, followed later by sunburn. The most common phototoxins are *psoralin* compounds, which are found in limes, lemons, celery, and parsnips. I recall one particularly surprising case of psoralin photoxicity: a woman who developed painful, large blisters which appeared on the backs of her hands after she had cut limes in the midday sun to make key-lime pie!

Another phototoxic substance is the wonderful fragrance from the peel of a specific orange grown in southern France and Italy called "oil of bergamot". I quite frequently see patients with brown skin stains as if liquid had dripped from behind their ear down their neck. This is the result of a photodermatitis called *berloque dermatitis* (from the French word meaning "pendant"), which occurs when someone applies perfume before sunbathing. These dark stains can persist for many months and often require medical treatment to lighten them. To avoid this problem, I advise my patients to apply all perfumes and colognes to the skin *under* their clothes, and not to any exposed skin.

Other phototoxic substances you may come across are *furocoumarins*. These are found in many foods and drinks, such as figs, greens, tonic drinks with quinine, and some cyclamates used in calorie-free drinks, as well as in some perfumes.

Photoallergies

A *photoallergy* is a specific immune reaction that occurs only in *certain* people after they have been exposed several times to the offending substance and then sunbathed or used a tanning bed. Even a small amount of the substance can cause a red, scaly or blistering eruption when the person sunbathes. The rash usually begins over 12 hours after exposure.

A photoallergic reaction is very individual. Some of the medicines and other products that can cause such a sensitivity are listed in Table 3.

Chloasma

Chloasma (also called "melasma" or "mask of pregnancy") is a dark brown, splotchy staining most frequently on the cheeks, but also on the forehead, upper lip, and neck. Chloasma develops slowly in about one-third of women taking oral contraceptives, fewer women taking hormonal replacement medications, and two-thirds of women during their second or third trimester of pregnancy. Some women, especially those with darker skin, are genetically predisposed to suffer from the condition. The cause is the combination of estrogen hormones and sun exposure. The dark skin stains fade gradually after delivery or when hormone medications are discontinued, provided the skin is well protected from the sun. Daily use of prescription bleaching creams containing hydroquinone can accelerate fading from about one year to three months.

Premature aging and precancers

If these consequences of sunburn and photosensitivity have not worried you enough, you need to accept the fact that the sun really does cause your skin to age prematurely. There is no such thing as a safe tan! Tanning is actually the visible evidence of damage to the skin. This is the same damage that causes skin cancer, premature wrinkling and aging, skin rashes and also decreased skin immunity.

Exposing your skin to the sun damages your collagen and elastic tissue. Especially on your face the sun damage produces many tiny wrinkles and deepens all your expression lines.

The sun also causes freckles, dark spots especially on the face, chest and hands (these are often misnamed "liver spots" or "age spots" although they actually have nothing to do with the liver nor with natural aging), as well as mottled discoloration and sometimes little white spots in sun-exposed areas. The sun is responsible for that rough, leathery appearance of skin (often seen on the necks of fishermen and farm laborers) as well as small, rough patches of skin which can be actual precancers (known as "actinic keratoses").

It is well worth remembering that at the end of your vacation your tan will quickly fade, but your skin will carry a permanent record of damage. Today's tan is tomorrow's wrinkle!

Skin cancer

Sun exposure also causes skin cancer. Conversely, the number of skin cancers that can be prevented by avoiding sun exposure is enormous. In the United States, one in every six Americans will suffer from skin cancer at some time in their lives, and one out of every three cancers diagnosed is a skin cancer.

Here's a frightening statistic: in America over the past decade, the number of skin cancers and deaths due to skin cancers has increased more than that of any other type of cancer (save the increase in deaths due to lung cancer in smoking women). The information below may not be pleasant but it's very important: it may help you or someone you care about.

There are three kinds of skin cancer: *basal cell carcinoma* (the most common type which enlarges but does not spread throughout the body), *squameous cell carcinoma* (which can spread), and the potentially deadly *melanoma*. All these are described in detail in Chapter 6.

A most shocking result of our sun-loving lifestyles is that the number of melanomas has doubled in each of the past five decades. Today, people are twice as likely to suffer from melanoma as 10 years ago. Malignant melanoma is currently the most common cancer in women between 25 and 29 years old, and more than one-fourth of all melanomas occur in people who are younger than 40. Just one severe case of sunburn can double your lifetime chance of developing melanoma, and two severe cases of sunburn in childhood or adolescence can triple that risk! If a family member has had a melanoma, the risk also increases.

Because in its early stages it is treatable and because it can spread quickly throughout the body very early, it is very important to see a doctor regularly if you have many moles, and as soon as any new dark spot appears anywhere on your body, especially if you have fair skin.

Decreased immunity

Your skin is your first layer of protection from the environment. Chapter 2 discussed how your skin has an immune system of its own – the Langerhan's cells. These capture foreign substances and organisms to present them to the immune system deeper in the skin and in the blood.

It is known that after exposure to UV light, the number of Langerhan's cells markedly decreases and can even disappear completely, making us far more susceptible to skin infection. When you suffer sunburn you compound the problem. Not only are your immune cells depleted, but the blistering of acute sunburn breaks down the skin, making infection more likely.

Fortunately, in most healthy people, the back-up provided by our immune system fights any invading organism. But for someone with an immune system weakened by medication (such as chemotherapy or steroids) or by disease (such as lymphoma or AIDS), the breakdown of the outer immune defence can be very serious.

When the immune system is weakened, the body is less able to deal with abnormal cells. A strong and healthy immune system successfully fights aberrant cell growths every day, killing off any abnormality immediately. But an immune system that is damaged by sun exposure is less able to perform its task.

The sun actually activates viral infections. About one in three people experiences a "fever blister" or "cold sore" on their lip, caused by the virus *herpes simplex,* after being on the beach. A recent study of people with recurrent fever blisters shows that if they use a sunscreen of at least SPF 15 (I recommend SPF 25–30) before sun exposure, not one fever blister will occur. People who are susceptible to cold sores should apply sunscreen to their lips at regular intervals when outdoors, especially after swimming, eating or drinking. It is easier for women to follow this advice than men since lipstick acts as a partial sunblock. There are also lip applicators designed specially for men.

Ultraviolet light can also activate other viruses. Most seriously, it has been confirmed that direct sunlight can activate the HIV virus which causes AIDS. This means that if an individual is already infected with HIV, the disease may progress more rapidly if that person is exposed to sun.

Eye damage

You realize by now that sunlight can particularly damage the delicate skin around your eyes and can cause skin cancer, especially on the lower lids which are more exposed to the sun than the upper lids. Also, exposure to direct sunlight can damage your eyes themselves. The most significant consequence later in life is the increased incidence of cataracts. These are the painless clouding of the eye's lens that can, in many cases, cause substantial loss of vision if they are not surgically removed.

Although cataracts do occur with normal aging and because of certain diseases or trauma, too much sunlight increases the risk of cataracts and can also make early cataracts worse. Worldwide each year, cataracts blind 12–15 million people and seriously impair the vision of another 18–30 million. Fortunately, the surgical removal of cataracts is a relatively routine and uncomplicated operation with very minimal risk.

Excessive exposure to the sun without sunglasses can also actually cause a sudden, painful sunburn to the eye, called *keratoconjunctivitis*. This usually occurs several hours after UV exposure and temporarily prevents the sufferer comfortably opening the eyes. Medication is needed and the person must wear an eye patch.

Chronic UV exposure may also contribute to an abnormal growth on the eyeball, called a *pterygium*. These growths should be surgically removed if vision is affected.

Who is at risk? Everyone!

No one is safe from sun damage! You learned your Sun-Sensitivity Skin Type in Chapter 3. You suffer an increased risk if your skin is Type I or II – that is if you are of Scottish, Irish, Scandinavian, or northern European descent and have fair skin that burns easily but does not tan. Especially at risk are people who have freckles, blond, red or light-brown hair, and blue, green or gray eyes.

Anyone with a lot of moles has an extra risk of getting skin cancer from sun exposure, as does anyone with a previous skin cancer or a family history of any type of skin cancer.

Skin cancers are less common in darker-skinned people, particularly southern Europeans such as Italians, Spaniards, Greeks and Portuguese people who have Types II, III or IV skin. Asians, Hispanics and Indians with Type V skin and sub-Saharan Africans with Type VI skin are less at risk because their skin contains more of the protective pigment melanin.

But even if you have darker skin, you need to limit sun exposure. A new, dark mole on *anyone* (especially on a palm or sole) can be a skin cancer and should be examined by a doctor immediately.

The closer you get to the equator and the higher the altitude, the greater the radiation-risk and increased risk from the sun. Fair-skinned people who live in northern regions must be especially cautious when they go away to southern climates. Going south in the winter or skiing in the strong snow-reflected sun can result in a very severe sunburn.

Children especially must be protected from the sun, not only from daily exposure in the summer months but also when on vacation at other times. Statistics show that about one-half of a person's life-time exposure to the sun is before 18. A single, blistering sunburn in a child doubles the risk of skin cancer as an adult. In fact, if a child is well protected from the sun until he or she is 12 years old, more than 80 percent of the risk of skin cancer as an adult is eliminated!

Up to two-thirds of our lifetime sun exposure is involuntary. That is, it occurs during everyday activities such as driving, gardening, walking to the car or to work. Not only sand (which reflects 17 percent of the sun's radiation), water, and snow (which reflects 85 percent), but also concrete pavements or sidewalks can act as natural "reflectors", increasing our exposure to ultraviolet rays.

Keep in mind that even on cloudy or hazy days, up to 80 percent of the sun's ultraviolet radiation is not filtered! If you play a lot of outdoor sports or you work outdoors, it is essential to wear protective clothing, a hat, and a sunscreen.

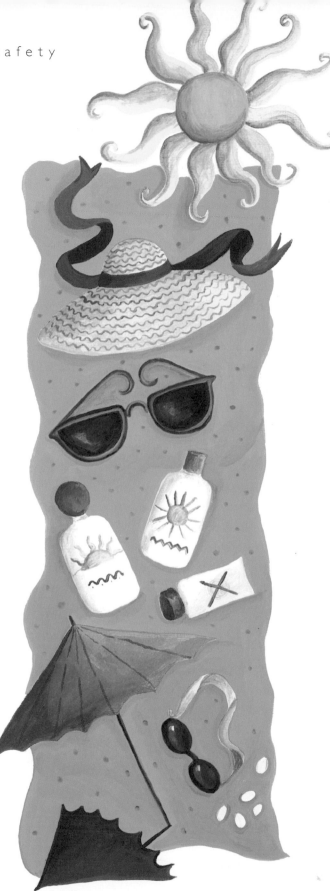

Protect yourself from damaging sunrays : the basic rules

These are the basic rules that really do help to protect you:

1 Don't roast yourself

However tempting it might be, don't ever lie in the sun. If you do for short periods, take all the proper precautions discussed in this chapter. And always stay near trees for shade or an umbrella (preferably dark and tightly woven). Do remember that indoor "palefaces" who quick-roast themselves in the sun on a two-week vacation can measurably increase their risk of skin cancer..

2 Beware of hidden sun

Guard against passive exposure to the sun. Experts emphasize that it's the 10 and 20 minute spurts of unprotected sun exposure – going to work, taking your children to school, running errands in your lunch break, for example – that take their destructive toll on skin over the years.

3 Mind the midday madness

Avoid the sun as much as possible during the peak radiation hours of 10am–4pm. Follow the "Shadow Rule": If your shadow is shorter than you are, the sun is directly overhead and you should be indoors. Arrange your children's play-time so that they are indoors during these hours.

4 Always use protective sunscreen

Use a protective sunscreen all year round (see below). Apply liberally 15–30 minutes before exposure and re-apply every two hours when you are in the sun.

5 Keep the cover on

Always keep covered up! Wear a wide-brimmed hat, long-sleeved shirts and trousers (pants) or a beach robe in the direct sun. Lightweight, lightly colored, tightly woven cotton clothing is best for sun protection (they reflect some UVA and B) and for comfort. Be aware that loosely woven or see-through fabrics do not protect from the sunlight, and that wet, clinging bathing suits are often transparent to harmful ultraviolet radiation. Generally, when fabrics are wet, their protection is decreased.

6 Shelter the kids

Keep your children under wraps. The tender skin of babies and young children is especially vulnerable to sunburn. Keep very young infants off the beach and older babies covered up in the shade. Begin using sunscreen on children at six months, then allow sun exposure only with moderation. Your young children won't know the difference in their early years, but they will certainly benefit from your sun-care for the rest of their lives.

7 Sunglasses are cool

Always protect your eyes! Wear dark sunglasses whenever you are outside in sunlight. When you're buying sunglasses, make sure you spot the ones that give the protection you need. (See helpful tips below.)

8 Tanning salons

Tanning salons should really be avoided. Some salons promise a "safe" tan from UVA, the "black light" of UVA rays alone, but this is not true. You learned above that UVA radiation causes damage to the deep layer of your skin, destroying the structural proteins collagen and elastin and impairing the immune system of the skin, enhancing cancer risk. Furthermore, it is this UVA which activates phototoxicities and also photoallergies.

If you are taking even a common medication that is photosensitizing, you could get a severe burn from just a short exposure to UVA. More-over, tanning lamps often emit doses of UVA far higher than is found in sunlight – and some may also emit UVB rays.

9 There are supplements

Some vitamin and mineral supplements available from health stores do help to protect your skin from the sun's radiation. They work by helping your body's natural protective systems kill the activated "free radicals" that form when the ultraviolet light hits your skin.

Taking vitamin E (400 IU per day of d- -toco-pheryl acetate or succinate) is like having a sunscreen of about SPF4. (Check with your pedi-atrician to see if a small dosage is recommended for your child.)

Also, the essential trace mineral selenium decreases skin damage after sun exposure. I have found that an adult with a history of excessive sun exposure would benefit from taking 50 to 200 micrograms a day of selenium, which can be purchased from health food stores in the form of L-selenomethione or brewer's yeast. Children under 10 years old should not be given selenium since many trace minerals may alter dental enamel during the period of tooth formation, increasing susceptibility to decay.

What sunscreen should I choose?

It should reassure you to know that sunscreens are classified as over-the-counter drugs, not merely cosmetics. That means that all ingredients in each preparation have undergone testing to demonstrate their safety and effectiveness. Each particular sunscreen formulation must also be checked prior to sale to demonstrate its sun protection factor (SPF).

Interestingly, the sunscreen ingredients accepted as effective by regulatory bodies differ a little from country to country. This has resulted in some truly effective sunscreen compounds commonly in use for years in the United Kingdom and Europe having only recently been accepted by the American Food and Drug Administration (FDA) (and only in very specific formulations) and others have yet to be accepted.

There is further variance in sunscreens because the method of measuring SPF differs somewhat in the UK and in Europe from the US. In addition, because UVA protection has only recently been recognized as important, a system that accurately assesses a sunscreen's UVA protection has yet to be designed. A sunscreen's SPF refers, therefore, only to the degree of UVB protection.

Don't be deterred by confusion regarding sunscreening capabilities, nor by the large number of products available. Just follow these tips to help you to make an educated choice.

Sun Protection Factor

Basically, the higher the SPF, the more sun protection you get. The SPF tells how much longer it would take to get a sunburn when protected by a sunscreen as opposed to being unprotected. For example, if you would naturally burn after 20 minutes of unprotected sun exposure, with application of a sunscreen of SPF15, you would suffer the same degree of burn after 15 x 20 minutes which equals five hours. That is, a sunscreen of SPF15 is meant to reduce to one fifteenth the amount of sun-damage caused over a given period of unprotected exposure.

As a dermatologist, I recommend a minimum sunscreen of SPF15 at all times and an SPF of 25–30 when you're exposed to bright sun, particularly on your face and hands (which suffer the most frequent exposure). An SPF of 4–8 gives very little protection. Application of an SPF of more than 30 is not necessary and, in fact, can sometimes be detrimental, since the additional chemicals in these preparations may actually be irritating to the skin.

Sunscreen types

There is a bewildering array of sunscreens available. Sunscreen ingredients are of two basic types: 1) physical, which block all UV radiation because they act as an actual, physical barrier refracting the light away from your skin's surface; and 2) chemical, which absorb certain specific wavelengths of the UV range.

Physical sunscreens

An example of a physical sunscreen is the familiar white zinc oxide coating that has long been the hallmark of the lifeguard's nose. Although these "sunblocks" are very effective, they are usually thick, often greasy and may cause pimples or prickly heat as well as stains on clothes.

Recently, however, new preparations of physical sunscreens have been formulated using tiny, "micronized" crystals of titanium dioxide that do not give a chalky appearance and actually help absorb oil from greasy skin. Also, new physical sunblocks are now made in flesh tones for cosmetically conscious adults and in bright, vivid colors for children (who really enjoy painting their faces as they protect their noses, cheeks, foreheads, ears and lips).

Chemical sunscreens

There are more than 20 different compounds that the American FDA recognizes as safe and effective ingredients of chemical sunscreens. The most common are: 1) para-aminobenzoic acid (PABA) and PABA derivatives (known as esters, such as padimate-O and padimate-A); 2) cinnamates; 3) salicylates (all three types absorb only UVB); 4) benzophenones (such as oxybenzone which absorbs primarily UVA); and 5) anthranilides, which absorb UVA as well as UVB.

PABA and PABA esters are the most effective chemical sunscreens for absorbing UVB but unfortunately they tend to induce a high incidence of allergy. This allergy can appear as a rash, or can manifest itself as a sunburn (sometimes rendering the cause of the redness ambiguous).

If you are allergic to PABA, you may also be allergic to the "-caine" group of anesthetics (including benzocaine and cocaine, but not lidocaine), to certain hair dyes (those containing paraphenylene diamine), and to sulfonamide antibiotics – so take care! PABA sunscreens have the further disadvantage that they can stain clothing, especially if you put your clothes on before they are completely absorbed.

The most effective sunscreen for absorbing UVA is avobenzone or Parsol 1789, which is relatively new to the United States but has been accepted for a long time in Europe. At this time in the United States, avobenzone is available in only two commercial formulations. In choosing your sunscreen, it is most important to be certain you have a product that gives you protection to both UVA and UVB.

Waterproof and water-resistant

"Water-resistant" sunscreens wash off after 40 minutes of swimming or perspiring with exercise; "waterproof" sunscreens last up to 80 minutes. The sunscreen you choose should definitely be waterproof. All rub off on clothing and towels, so be sure to re-apply sunscreen at least every one to two hours, especially if you are perspiring or swimming regularly. Remember, when wet your skin absorbs more UV because its outer layer becomes more transparent and when swimming there are reflected rays from the water's surface.

Gel, lotion, cream or ointment?

The choice of physical form of sunscreen that you apply is entirely your personal taste. If you have a tendency to an oily complexion or acne, you might prefer a sunscreen with micronized titanium dioxide which is not greasy, or an alcohol-based or gel sunscreen. Men usually prefer alcoholic or gel sunscreens since they resemble after-shave cologne. Alcohols and gels, however, can irritate dry skin. Cream-based sunscreens, on the other hand, moisturize the skin, but wash off more easily. Your face should have the highest SPF protection, and often your face is oily, while your hands and body are dry. For this reason, you might even feel more comfortable using one formulation of sunscreen on your face (for example, alcohol-based) and another on your body (for example, cream-based). You might seek the advice of your dermatologist on this or experiment yourself to see what works best for you.

Sunscreen guidelines

Because sunscreen is so important in helping you maintain a youthful and healthy skin, I would suggest that you consult a dermatologist if you are uncertain as to which brand or formulation to choose. My own line of Longévité® skincare products (see page 128), for example, provides several formulations. Table 4, below, gives a number of handy guidelines.

Table 4

Sunscreen Guidelines

1   Choose a sunscreen of at least SPF 25 to 30, especially in bright sunlight.

2   Be sure that the sunscreen you use is water-proof, particularly if you swim or perspire a lot.

3   Be sure your sunscreen protects against UVA as well as UVB.

4   Suit your skin. Choose a gel or alcohol sunscreen formulation for your face if you have oily skin; use a moisturizing cream, lotion or ointment formulation if your skin is dry.

5   Reapply your sunscreen every 1½ to 2 hours when outdoors.

Be careful!

Wearing sunscreen is not a licence to expose yourself to the sun for hours on end. You still need to be careful. If you are wearing a sunscreen that protects better against UVB, for example, the fact that it protects you from burning may tempt you to stay in the sun for longer. In the process, you could suffer much more and deeper UVA damage than if you had used no sunscreen at all!

Choosing the right sunglasses

Always wear sunglasses when you are outdoors and exposed to solar radiation. Your eyes need the protection. So, incidentally, does the skin around your eyes, which is especially delicate and susceptible to sun damage. Wrinkles are a factor, too. Without protective sunglasses, sunlight makes us squint giving us both "crow's feet" wrinkles alongside our eyes and extra wrinkles across our forehead.

Sunglasses come in all shapes and sizes. More importantly for our purposes, they also come with lenses of very differing quality and capability. Here are a few tips on what you might look for to best protect your eyes.

Look carefully at the labels and always buy dark sunglasses that are labelled "Blocks all UVB" or "Blocks 95 percent UVB". Labels stating "Special Purpose" mark glasses designed for skiing and other high exposure activities that block at least 99 percent of UVB.

Labels stating "General Purpose" are made for daily wear and mark glasses that block 95 percent of UVB. Labels stating only "Blocks UV", without an indicated degree of absorption, may

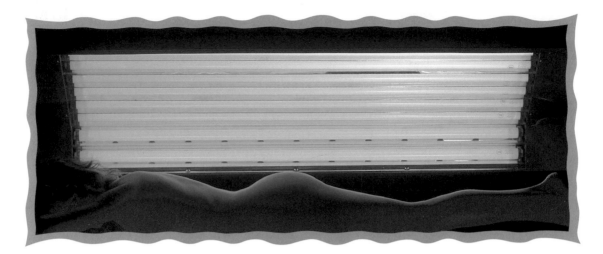

not give enough protection. Labels that state "Cosmetic", the least protective group, let in up to 30 percent of UVB light!

Do not go to tanning salons! The UVA rays damage your skin and can cause serious burns.
Science Photo Library, London

Watch out for the fact that neither the color of the lens nor the darkness of the tint indicates how well the sunglasses filter UV light. Darker lenses that have no UVB filter are actually more detrimental than wearing no sunglasses at all, since darker lenses cause more dilation of the pupil so that more UVB radiation reaches the eye's lens.

Polarized lenses reduce reflection and glare but do not absorb UV unless so indicated. *Photochromatic* lenses change color in sunlight and may filter UV light. Clear UV-absorbing coatings are also available for prescription glasses and can be applied to glasses or goggles used for skiing, high altitude flying and other outdoor sports.

Always make sure that your glasses fit properly. Glasses that slip down your nose, even fractionally, can let unfiltered sunlight reach your eyes.

When in doubt, ask for advice. You will find that the price of glasses varies not with their protective effectiveness but more with their role as fashion objects. Make certain that you are buying more than just a fashionable frame, and that your sunglass lenses effectively protect your eyes from a very high percentage of harmful ultraviolet radiation.

Self-tanners are fine...

The only "safe" tan is the tan obtained from a bottle! Effective self-tanning creams contain the chemical *dihydroxyacetone,* which reacts with the keratin protein in the outer layers of skin to dye the skin brown. (Be careful! Dihydroxyacetone darkens all keratin protein, including hair and wool.)

This type of self-tanner is perfectly safe and can give the tan you desire if applied properly and uniformly. There are many formulas which give different shades of tan. The consistency of the cream or lotion also varies – self-tanner must be applied evenly to prevent splotchiness. Quite a few products are good, so experiment with several brands until you find one that you prefer.

Because your skin loses its outer layer of cells each day, you may need to apply self-tanner daily to maintain the skin color you want. Be sure to wash your hands immediately after applying a self-tanner or your palms will stain dark brown.

If you want a "darker" tan, just apply self-tanner more than once a day. Keep in mind that this tan does not protect you from the sun in any way! You must still use a sunscreen whenever you are outside.

Some self-tanning creams contain the natural amino acid, tyrosine. Although tyrosine is the molecule from which your natural pigment, melanin, is made, I have not seen evidence that it can be absorbed by the skin or that it promotes the production of your own melanin.

... not so, tanning accelerators!

Stay away from tanning accelerators, which come in the form of creams or pills. They can be dangerous! They most commonly contain a derivative of the compound psoralin. A tanning pill developed in Germany but not permitted in the United States consists of a combination of B-carotene and the carotenoid canthaxantin. All tanning accelerators when taken or applied photosensitize to UVA rays and accelerate the damage done by UVA.

In other words, tanning accelerators accelerate the premature aging of your skin, they decrease your skin's immunity, and they accentuate photo-toxicities and photoallergies. The oral forms of tanning accelerator can be especially harmful because they speed up damage to unprotected eyes, with the risk of such damage continuing for several days after use.

After taking the canthaxantin capsules, many patients complain of difficulty with adapting their eyesight to the dark. On examination, 75 percent of users were found to have minor abnormalities of their eyes' retinal pigment.

These products should be avoided unless prescribed by a physician for treatment of a specific disease. If they are used, protective precautions (including wearing UV protective glasses for at least two days after use) must be taken, as directed.

It's never too late!

Let's face it – if we're honest most of us would admit that they had not practised the best of "sun-habits" over the years. In the past nobody had the knowledge that is available today. Indeed, many people grew up with the belief that the sun, which felt so good, was also good for our health. No matter what your past practices have been, don't be discouraged by what you have read in this chapter! Everybody can start taking the proper precautions immediately. And this book will show you how to treat, and even reverse, some of the ill effects of your past sunbathing sessions.

Do enjoy your travelling and your outdoor sports. But always protect yourself and especially your children from the sun's dangerous ultraviolet rays. Whenever you are in the sun, do as the Australians do: "Slip on a beach robe, slap on a hat, and slop on sunscreen."

By doing this, you will keep healthy and stay looking young. You will learn a simple and effective program of lifetime skin fitness that treats your skin with the care that it really deserves!

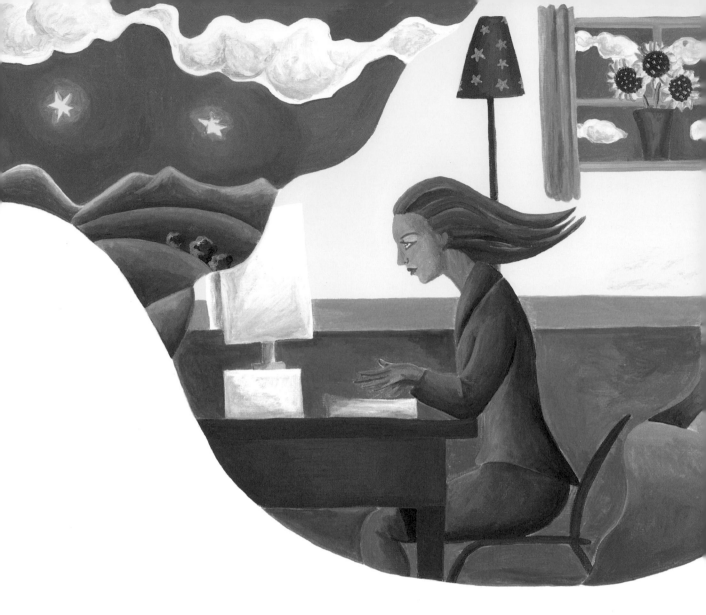

Your "Indoor Skin"

Have you ever heard of an "indoor environmentalist"? Most people associate the environment with the "great outdoors" and the "wonders of
nature". On the contrary, our own "environments" are increasingly
indoors, and increasingly "unnatural". Whether at home or at the office,
your skin suffers in special ways from the indoor environment with its
closed atmosphere and surrounding work materials. How do you recognize actual or potential irritants? How can you protect your skin from daily
damage by the indoor surroundings you take for granted? How can you
correct or at least improve your indoor environment?

City skin

Today, more than three-quarters of us live or work in cities. Cities give us economic and intellectual stimuli, energy, cultural excitement and convenient contact with friends and colleagues. But as we gravitate increasingly to urban areas, our health, and particularly our skin, can suffer.

Any fresh air indoors?

Buildings used to be designed with systems to assure constant air flow volume for heating, cooling and ventilation. Today's "energy efficient" structures are quite different. New buildings are tightly sealed, with recirculated air. Internal sources (lights, machines) provide extra heat, and air delivery rates are varied to maintain temperature, not necessarily to meet air quality needs. In large buildings, fresh air supplies are frequently reduced to a minimum to conserve energy.

The indoor Sahara

The average urban worker is indoors 90 percent of the day. Indoor environments dry the skin – with excessive heat in winter and excessive air conditioning in summer. This is quite simple to rectify. First, turn down the heating or air conditioning, especially at home. There's no reason to roast in winter or freeze in summer! Secondly, install a humidifier, and be sure to keep it clean to prevent bacteria build-up in the water! The simplest, and least costly "humidifier" is an open pan of water near the radiator or air conditioner (which helps preserve wooden furniture as well!). If you work in a closed office space, be sure always to apply a moisturizer after you wash your hands or face.

Deskside pollution

Your office environment contains potentially hazardous air pollutants! The most significant indoor contaminant (in countries where it's not banned) is cigarette smoke, accounting for up to 30–40 percent of indoor pollution. If you smoke, you can spare your own skin and that of your fellow workers by stopping. In fact, prohibiting smoking in sealed buildings very significantly improves the health of all occupants.

Indoor contaminants from outdoor sources, such as car exhaust or dust from construction, are second on the list. These are drawn into buildings through intake vents. A simple filtration system can be helpful in reducing such pollutants. If you or your co-workers smell fumes or experience symptoms such as headaches or stinging eyes, it may be worth investigating.

The third most common contaminants are chemicals in the air or on surfaces. Chemicals cause over 90 percent of industrial allergic reactions! Your office, work place, or home may contain a number of potential irritants and allergens; finding the offender can call for some good detective work. The most common chemical irritants are volatile organic compounds from adhesive, tile, vinyl wall coverings and furniture.

Formaldehyde is the most common, present in many fabrics, paints, carpets, draperies and cleaning agents and released into the air by many copying machines. If you notice skin symptoms such as redness, itching, swelling, rashes, or blemishes (which can arise either shortly after contacting an offending substance or a day or two later), or if you have a sudden onset of eye irritation, rhinitis (nose inflammation), headache, or rash after your office or home was painted, new carpets or draperies were installed, or a floor was polished, formaldehyde may be the culprit. If you come into skin contact with a chemical (unless instructed otherwise), wash thoroughly as soon as possible. (Sometimes the chemical container lists precautions and instructions for removal after contact.) If you notice a rash or skin reaction, see your dermatologist.

From glue to flowers

There are many potential allergens in our indoor environments, particularly synthetic resins found in glues, solvents, and insulating materials. Specific professions have particular hazards: beauticians or hairdressers work with hair tints and permanent solutions; construction workers use fuels, lubricants, and cements; chefs, bartenders, and bakers handle juices (notable allergens are pineapple, orange, and lemon) and spices (cayenne pepper (capsicum), cinnamon, cloves, nutmeg, and vanilla are particular culprits); printers touch acrylics, epoxies, and ink. Anybody can suffer skin allergies from touching Japanese lacquer, ivory, or bamboo furniture.

Pressure or rubbing with repetitive motions causes irritations and blisters, and can also stimulate or worsen an allergic reaction. For example, working repeatedly with scissors, paper clips, letter openers and kitchen utensils, especially if the skin is moist, can cause rashes on areas of the skin touching these implements if you are allergic to nickel. Wearing rubber gloves while doing housework can protect you. (Your dermatologist can test you for nickel allergy and can show you how to test objects for nickel content.)

Flowers and plants are wonderful to see and smell but not necessarily to touch! Chrysanthemums and dahlias have the same "poison" as poison ivy; orchids, primrose, tulips, daffodils, sunflowers, lilacs, begonias and ivy can all cause allergic skin reactions in many people.

Touch and wash

As a dermatologist, I frequently see patients with skin problems caused by irritants and allergens in their indoor environments. Many facial rashes, including acne, occur because an individual touches his or her face after having handled seemingly harmless common objects such as formaldehyde-rich newsprint or naphthalene-containing copying paper. (Pesticides are particularly irritating and can exacerbate acne, so if you're working in your garden, wash your hands as soon as you step indoors!)

Facial rashes, especially around the eyes, are more often caused by hand-transmission of irritants than by makeup! Washing hands with a mild cleanser or soap after touching an irritant or allergen can help prevent any reaction.

Allergy or irritation?

Allergies and irritations are different (as discussed in Chapter 7). An *irritation* occurs in everyone who comes in contact with an offending substance, though some more sensitive people might react to lower concentrations or fewer contacts. (If concentrated formaldehyde were applied to anybody's fingers or face, for example, he or she would develop a dry, flaky, red, painful rash. Very sensitive skins could be irritated by a trace of formaldehyde, just touching a newspaper or even being in a room with new curtains.)

An *allergy*, on the other hand, is a genetic predisposition. The person must already have been exposed to the allergen at least once, and the allergy might show itself on the second, tenth, or ten-thousandth contact!

Some people are particularly susceptible:
- In general, women are more sensitive than men because their skin is thinner and less oily.
- Younger skin is more sensitive than older skin.
- Sensitivity runs in families. If close relatives have hay fever or asthma, you are more likely to be sensitive.

Sick buildings?

Because of non-specific symptoms at times experienced by workers in sealed buildings, some environmental scientists have talked about the existence of so-called "sick building syndrome." In my opinion, there is no single "sick building syndrome". The fact that some buildings have contaminants or even infectious organisms not easily cleared from their "circulatory systems" is a reality, however, and can be a significant problem. To confirm that a problem exists, certain questions should be asked:
- Are symptoms specifically related to time spent in a particular building, or in part of that building?

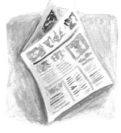

- Do symptoms resolve when the person is not in the building?
- Do symptoms recur seasonally or in relation to heating and cooling?
- Have fellow workers noted similar complaints?

Each case must be addressed individually so that offending causes can be properly evaluated and corrected, and any recurrence prevented.

Flying high

The plane is the ultimate "closed environment." The airline passenger is exposed to super-dry, recirculated air. We are all increasingly frequent fliers, so how do we best protect our skin?

The most damaging aspect of a plane's indoor environment is dryness – to skin, eyes, lips, and hair. Even the air of a sealed office building is moist compared to a plane cabin in which the humidity can be as low as 2 percent! Your body can lose up to 1 quart (.95 litre) more water per day in a plane than on land.

Everyone drinks on planes not just out of habit or boredom, but because they are thirsty. Avoid excessive alcohol, as it dehydrates and encourages jet lag. I recommend you drink at least one glass of non-sparkling mineral water or orange juice per hour in flight.

To save your skin from the extreme dryness, take toiletries and cosmetics in your carry-on luggage. Especially on a long flight, you will want to complete your normal morning routine (described in Chapter 8) before you arrive. If possible, use your own cleanser rather than commercial soaps. Always apply moisturizer *immediately* after washing even your hands.

If your lips become dry, apply a moisturizing lip balm (even your lip sunscreen or a chapstick will do) or petroleum jelly. Just as when you are outdoors in winter, avoid licking your lips: saliva is an irritant and dries the lips.

If you wear contact lenses, consider removing them in flight, especially if you are sleeping. Hard contact lenses, in particular, might scratch the surface of your eyes, which are made drier than usual by the cabin's extreme dryness. Everyone should keep natural tears or eye drops on hand in flight. Any small particle in your eye is potentially more irritating when the eye surface is dry.

One last tip: eat lightly – preorder a "special meal" of vegetables or fruit. Exercise: do several sets of "Pressometrics" from my book, *Thin Thighs For Life,* to slim your thighs and your arms; rotate your ankles and wiggle your toes at least every half-hour while you are awake; take walks up and down the aisle to boost your circulation.

Smoke versus the smoker

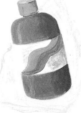

Of all smokers who start smoking in adolescence and continue throughout their lives, half will succumb to a fatal tobacco-caused disease before the age of 70, losing, on average, 22 years of their life expectancy!

In the United States, cigarette smoking is the *leading* cause of preventable, premature death. As more and more women smoke, so their incidence of heart disease and lung cancer has increased – their death rate from lung cancer has increased by a factor of almost seven from 1950 until 1990 (with the death rate from breast cancer showing little change over the same period). Whatever its pleasures, smoking's consequences are most unpleasant: chronic cough, hoarseness, asthma, bronchitis, emphysema, lung cancer, cancers of the mouth, throat, esophagus and bladder (all of which can be fatal), and increased risk of heart attack and stroke!

If all of this isn't bad enough, smoking really does ruin your skin. Smokers have far more wrinkles than non-smokers. In fact, studies demonstrate that heavy smokers (of 20 or more cigarettes per day) are almost *five times* more likely to have prominent wrinkles than non-smokers! Smokers' skin quality is damaged by direct injury of the collagen and elastic tissue support, and smokers also unattractively pucker their lips to inhale, and squint from the irritating smoke in their eyes. Consequently, smokers have more wrinkles around their mouths and on their foreheads and cheeks than non-smokers, and more prominent "crow's feet" around their eyes.

Smokers' faces are pale, sallow, and gray, often with more tiny blood vessels (called *telangiectasia)* on the nose and cheeks. Smokers' skin is also thickened and leathery, similar to that seen on the sun-damaged skin of fishermen and farmers, indicating severe degradation of the elastic tissue. In a nutshell, smokers look unhealthy and prematurely aged!

But that's not all; it's more than cosmetic! Smokers have an increased risk of squamous cell skin cancer on the head and neck and an increased recurrence of this skin cancer after treatment. And smokers suffer from decreased wound healing. Indeed, 85 percent of the complications in healing after face-lift surgery occur in smokers, sometimes even causing permanent loss of skin color or scarring. Stopping smoking one month or more before surgery can reduce these complications, but not to the level of non-smokers. Many plastic surgeons will not perform a face-lift on any smoker!

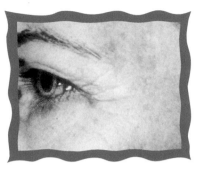

Smoking increases wrinkles: this 57-year-old woman does not smoke.

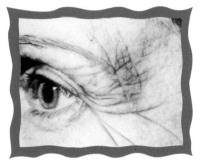

This wrinkled 51-year-old woman has smoked for many years.
Mayo Clinic Health Letter, January 1987

The decrease in healing capacity in all smokers is most probably caused by nicotine, which constricts blood vessels not only at the sites of wounds but in all skin, particularly in the fingers and toes. Nicotine stains fingers and teeth, and gives the breath a stale odor. And nicotine itself is a poison! A one pack per day cigarette smoker consumes 400mg of nicotine a week – enough to cause instant death if taken in one dose.

Passive smoking

Smokers harm more than themselves; they affect the lives of the non-smokers with whom they live and work. "Passive smoking" is a leading cause of preventable death in America (exceeded only by active smoking and alcohol). Non-smokers married to smokers have an increased risk of lung cancer by 30 percent. Passive smoking may account for as many as ten times the number of deaths from heart disease as lung cancer. Children whose parents smoke (especially if the mother smokes) have a higher prevalence of bronchitis, pneumonia, wheezing, coughing and middle ear disease.

Why does other people's smoke cause so much damage? "Mainstream smoke" (even filtered) inhaled by a smoker contains large-particle toxins that are deposited in the mouth and in the larger airways of the body. "Side-stream smoke" from a burning cigarette actually contains higher amounts of up to 4,000 dangerous compounds, of which more than 50 are carcinogenic. These compounds are in tiny particles which can be inhaled more deeply into the lungs and absorbed into the bloodstream to affect the entire body, including the skin.

Just quit!

Making the decision to give up smoking isn't easy. Smoking is an insidious and addictive habit that's very difficult to break. But is it worth all the harm it causes?

For a long life – and a great skin – a smoker can only benefit by stopping now!

Lumps and Bumps

This chapter should be taken seriously. It might not be a lot of fun to read, but it contains the sort of information that can be vital to the wellbeing of any individual. And it suggests simple practices that might save you and those you love a great deal of time and trouble. The information in this chapter is meant to raise your awareness of possible problems and to tell you something about your own body and what you might be able to observe from looking at your skin.

On no account should you attempt to diagnose yourself. Only a qualified doctor can do that! (Even doctors go to other doctors when they need to be examined and treated!)

There is no substitute for a periodic medical checkup, which should include regular visits to a qualified dermatologist. The recommended frequency of such examinations varies with the specific circumstances and should be discussed with your doctor.

That said, the more aware you are of your physical (and, for that matter, spiritual) self, the better you might be able to seek appropriate help and advice when it is needed.

- **All right! Take your clothes off!** Not right now, necessarily! But when you're alone and have the time. Make sure you have access to a full-length mirror (as well as a hand-held mirror so you can see your back).
- **Look and feel!** Look at your skin – carefully – in all its perfection and imperfection. Run your hands over its smoothness, and feel for any rough spots.
- **Record!** Have a notepad and pencil at the ready and make a brief note of what you observe. If you don't do this, it is surprisingly easy to forget!

What are you looking for?

Everyone has some little spots on their skin. Some are transient, some are permanent. As you look carefully at yourself, you may be surprised to see for the first time tiny red dots, or flat or raised brown moles. You are all usually quite aware of any new blemish on your face, but maybe now with your careful examination, you will feel small rough patches or tiny bumps or see discoloration that you did not notice previously.

This chapter is not meant to give a definitive diagnosis of every possible lump and bump on you skin. Rather, photographs and descriptions of some of the most common skin lesions are presented. If you have any rash or any new spot on your skin that persists for more than a few weeks, you should visit your dermatologist. He or she can easily treat any such spot, and it is always better to do so sooner rather than later, since some lesions can enlarge and should be treated cosmetically while they are small, and others might be of medical importance.

When is it necessary to see a dermatologist about a new mole? Just as women should check their breasts systematically and carefully for new lumps, so every person should check their skin routinely for new moles at least each month. Some moles are benign but unattractive, others might be early skin cancers. All are treatable if they are diagnosed early.

Removal of benign lesions is quick and painless, since it can be done with local anesthesia if necessary. Superficial lesions, such as skin tags or seborrheic keratoses, are cut with tiny surgical scissors or scraped with a surgical curette, then touched with an electric needle. Some deeper moles should be cut more deeply for removal or for a biopsy, often requiring a stitch. The healing from these procedures takes about one week on the face and two to three weeks on the body or arms or legs. Warts and actinic keratosis are usually initially treated by cryosurgery, that is, freezing the cells with liquid nitrogen. Some lesions are best treated by laser.

Your monthly self-examination

1 Stand in front of a full-length mirror with no clothes. Examine the front and back of your body thoroughly. Then look carefully at your sides and under your arms.

2 Bend your elbows and look at your upper and lower arms (both the inner and outer surfaces). Remove your rings and observe your palms and between the fingers.

3 Observe the fronts and backs of your legs carefully. Look at your soles and at the spaces between your toes.

4 Check your back and buttocks and other creases in your body carefully with a hand mirror.

5 Examine the back of your neck and behind your ears with a hand mirror. Touch your scalp and part your hair for a closer look at any lumps or scabs.

When to see a dermatologist about a mole

1 If the mole is new.

2 If the mole has changed in appearance, especially in color.

3 If the surrounding skin has changed, especially if it becomes red or swollen or if colored blemishes form next to the mole.

4 If the border of the mole is asymmetric, irregular, or indistinct.

5 If the mole has "weeping" pigmentation into the surrounding skin.

6 If the mole has many shades of color: red, light brown, dark brown.

7 If the mole is on the palm, sole, lip, or gums.

8 If the mole is larger than 0.55cm (¼ in).

9 If the mole is repeatedly irritated by friction with clothes (collar, necklace, belt, bra) or by your repeatedly touching it.

10 If the mole is itchy, tender, or painful.

11 If the mole becomes scaly or ulcerated, or if it becomes moist or bloody.

12 If you are bothered by the mole's appearance.

Moles (nevi) are collections of nevus cells derived from the pigment-producing melanocytes. Almost everyone has at least one nevus, which can be flesh-colored, brown or bluish-black. Some are flat *(junctional)*, some slightly elevated *(compound)*, and some dome-shaped *(dermal)*. Nevi occur in about one percent of all newborn babies; the number of nevi increases in childhood. The size and pigmentation may increase throughout life, especially during puberty, pregnancy, with oral estrogens such as the Pill, and after sun exposure. Although some women such as Elizabeth Taylor are known for their distinctive "beauty marks", many moles are unattractive or irritating, and others may change in appearance. These should be removed for microscopic examination.

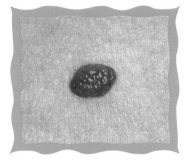

*The Skin Cancer
Foundation, New York*

Lentigines (singular: lentigo) are small, uniformly-colored, tan or brown, flat spots which are often difficult to distinguish from nevi. There are two types: *lentigo simplex* and *solar lentigo*. Lentigo simplex usually appears in childhood but can occur at any age, anywhere on the body, often on people with red or blonde hair. There is no connection with the sun. Solar lentigines (misnamed "liver spots", though they have nothing to do with the liver) are light brown spots mostly on the backs of the hands, chest, upper back, shoulders, and face. Although these are considered to be tell-tale signs of age, they are actually an unattractive result of sun-exposure. Lentigines do not become skin cancers. They can easily be removed using prescription bleaching agents or by cryosurgery.

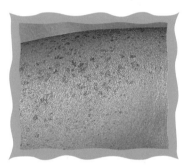

Science Photo Library, London

Dysplastic nevi are melanocytic nevi which are potentially dangerous since they have abnormal cells. The tendency to develop dysplastic nevi is hereditary, and there is usually a family history of melanoma. Some dysplastic nevi actually evolve into melanomas; even more significantly, people with dysplastic nevi have at least a ten times greater probability of developing a melanoma in their lifetimes than people who do not have any. Dysplastic nevi are recognized by their poorly defined border, irregularity in shape, and variegated, uneven color. Individuals with more than one hundred moles on their bodies almost always have several dysplastic nevi. Any mole which changes or which appears dysplastic should be biopsied for microscopic examination. Removing a mole does not in any way increase the risk of its spreading or changing.

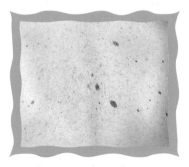

*Nia K. Terezakis, M.D.
Louisiana*

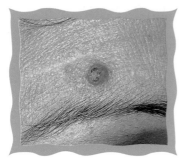

Science Photo Library, London

Basal cell carcinoma is by far the most common type of skin cancer. This usually appears as either a small, translucent lump (almost like a pimple that does not heal) on the face, ear, neck or hands, or as a reddish patch with a raised border, on the back or chest or hand. Basal cell carcinomas grow slowly but if left untreated they will begin to bleed, forming a grainy crust in the center as they enlarge at the edge. This type of cancer rarely spreads to other parts of the body, but it can spread locally below the skin, even to the bone. If treated early enough, there is only a minimal (and sometimes no) scar. If left untreated for a long period, the damage can be more extensive, and the scar that remains after removal will be larger.

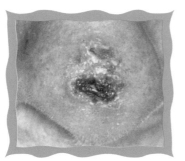

*The Skin Cancer
Foundation, New York*

Squameous cell carcinoma is the second most common form of skin cancer. It appears most often on sun-exposed areas such as the face, ears, upper chest and back, arms, and back of the hands. Pipe smokers often get squameous cell carcinomas on their lips or inside the mouth from having held their pipe between their teeth for long periods. These cancers at first appear simply as scaly patches that do not heal, growing to become ulcerated, red patches. They tend to grow faster than basal cell carcinomas. They invade not only locally, but they can also occasionally spread through the body, particularly if they were initially on the head and neck (especially the mouth, lips or scalp).

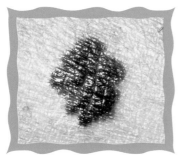

*The Skin Cancer
Foundation, New York*

Malignant melanoma is the deadliest form of skin cancer. There are four characteristic warning signs of melanoma – the "ABCD's": A for "asymmetry" such that one side of the mole is not round, but rather quite irregular; B for "border irregularity" with ragged, notched, blurred edges; C for "color not uniform" with shades of tan, brown, blue and black or red, mottled areas; and D for "diameter" larger than 6mm (¼in) (the size of a pencil eraser). A melanoma can appear anywhere on the body, not just in areas that have been exposed to the sun. Some melanomas develop from pre-existing dysplastic nevi; but some just seem to come from nowhere. Melanomas can be completely removed if they are caught in the initial stages, but they can spread rapidly throughout the body if they enlarge, so early diagnosis and prompt treatment are absolutely essential.

Seborrheic keratoses are slightly elevated, rough, scaly growths that appear "stuck" onto the surface of the skin. They are usually brown but can be skin-colored. They are often nicknamed "barnacles" or "stucco keratoses". Seborrheic keratoses are very common; almost everyone has at least one, and some individuals have more than one hundred! They can be found almost anywhere on the body, most prevalently on sun-exposed areas. Not only are seborrheic keratoses unsightly, but frequently they are itchy. Fortunately, they are benign and never become serious skin tumors. They are easily removed by curettage or by cryotherapy. These keratoses are superficial, so there is no residual scar. A biopsy is sometimes required to rule out a more serious skin tumor.

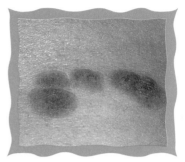

*Karen E. Burke Research
Foundation, New York*

Actinic keratoses (AKs) are flat or slightly raised, sometimes red, scaly patches which appear on the background of sun-damaged skin – especially on the face, the scalps of balding men, the backs of the hands, arms, chest and back. Since they are rough to the touch, AKs are often more easily diagnosed by feel than by observation. They are especially prevalent on fair-skinned people who continue to develop AKs even long after discontinuing sun exposure. AKs are pre-malignant skin growths that can develop into squameous cell carcinomas. They must therefore be treated straightaway, either by cryosurgery or chemotherapy using Effudex (5-fluorouracil) or Actinex (masoproco) cream. These creams cause the skin to become markedly inflamed for at least one week, but there is also some decrease in wrinkles as a bonus!

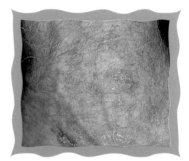

*The Skin Cancer
Foundation, New York*

Dermatofibromas are pink or dark brown nodules anywhere on the body, often on the legs. Dermatofibromas grow deeper into the skin and are firmer than moles. They can be identified by the so-called "dimple sign": when the surrounding skin is pinched, the dermatofibroma retracts. Dermatofibromas are actually scars composed of fibrous tissue that forms after a minor injury like an insect bite or infected hair follicle. Since they are benign and rarely cause symptoms of itching or discomfort, once they are identified, they can be ignored. However, since some dermatofibromas are unattractive and women often cut them when shaving their legs, they can easily be treated either conservatively with cryosurgery (to lighten and soften them) or by excision.

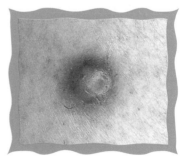

*Gloria F. Graham, M.D., North
Carolina*

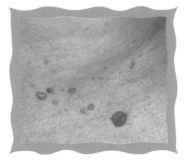

*Karen E. Burke Research
Foundation, New York*

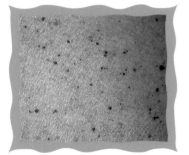

*Karen E. Burke Research
Foundation, New York*

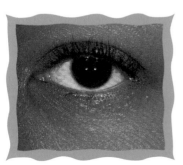

*Thomas P. Habif, M.D., New
Hampshire*

Skin tags (called *acrochordons* if they are small and *fibroephithelial* polyps if they are larger) are harmless, flesh-colored or light to dark brown extensions of the skin, attached on fine stalks most frequently on the eyelids, neck, shoulders, armpits, and groin. They usually appear with pregnancy or after the age of 40, especially in obese individuals, diabetics, and post-menopausal women. Multiple skin tags may be associated with intestinal polyps. If you have gastrointestinal symptoms and you do suddenly develop many skin tags, you should see your doctor. Although these small skin tags seldom cause problems, they are an unattractive nuisance and can often catch on jewelry. Larger ones can twist, resulting in bleeding and sometimes infection. They can be easily and painlessly removed by simple snipping and electrocautery.

Cherry angiomas are the small, smooth, red papules that occur in almost everyone after the age of 30. In some cases, a body can be dotted with hundreds of cherry angiomas, especially in older individuals.

Cherry angiomas are most common on the top half of the body, but they can occur anywhere. Cherry angiomas do not become malignant and are not dangerous. They are merely cosmetically unattractive, but larger ones do bleed if traumatized. The treatment is simple and takes only a few seconds; each angioma is just touched with an electric needle. Since the angioma is on the skin surface, there is no scarring. It is preferable to treat each angioma shortly after it first begins, since it will most probably enlarge with time.

Syringomas are tiny, flesh-colored or slightly yellow, firm papules that occur most frequently on the lower eyelids and sometimes on the fore-head, chest and abdomen. Syringomas are actually growths of the eccrine sweat glands which are completely benign. They are often mistaken for flat warts or pimples. They are more frequently found on women then men and are more common in Orientals. Syringomas first appear at puberty and can slowly become more numerous with age. Since syringomas are unattractive, they can easily be removed by superficial electrocautery or cryosurgery.

Warts (verruccae) are papilloma virus infections of the skin surface, and are most common in children. Warts mostly appear at sites of trauma, especially on the hands and nails (from nail biting). Smooth flat warts are frequent on the face and neck, projecting filiform warts can be anywhere on the body, and painful, deep plantar warts are common on the soles. Warts are easily recognized by their rough texture and the tiny black dots on the surface (which are actually blood vessels). Warts are spread simply by touch. A wart usually appears one to three months after contact, but this incubation time can be up to twelve months. Although about one-third of warts spontaneously disappear within six months, some warts can last a lifetime if they are left untreated.

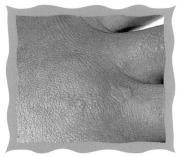

Science Photo Library, London

Mulluscum contagiosum is a viral infection of the skin characterized by a small, dome-shaped, flesh-colored papule with a central indented section. This was once almost exclusively a disease of children, but now this has left the classroom and entered the bedroom, often being spread by sexual contact. The lesions are grouped, usually on the face, trunk, underarms, and extremities in children, and in the pubic and genital areas in adults. The papules are spread by scratching or touching, especially on inflamed skin as atopic dermatitis or eczema. Although the lesions usually spontaneously clear in six to nine months, it is best to treat them before crops of new lesions spread. They can easily be removed by curettage or freezing.

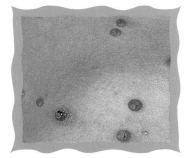

Science Photo Library, London

Herpes simplex (fever blisters or cold sores) are familiar infections of the skin caused by herpes virus type I or 2. Almost every child has one infection; 15 percent of the population suffer with recurrences, since the virus remains dormant in the nerves at the site of a previous infection. Trauma (sun exposure or chapping) and stress (including fever) can exacerbate flare-ups. The outbreak is preceded by discomfort or itching, then redness; finally clusters of tiny blisters filled with watery fluid appear. These change into pustules, then crusts which finally heal after eight to twelve days. The blister fluid and the crusts are infectious, so care must be taken not to scratch them and especially not to touch others. Recurrences are partially controlled with the prescription medication acyclovir (ointment or tablets).

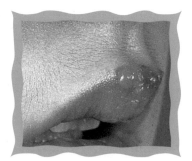

Science Photo Library, London

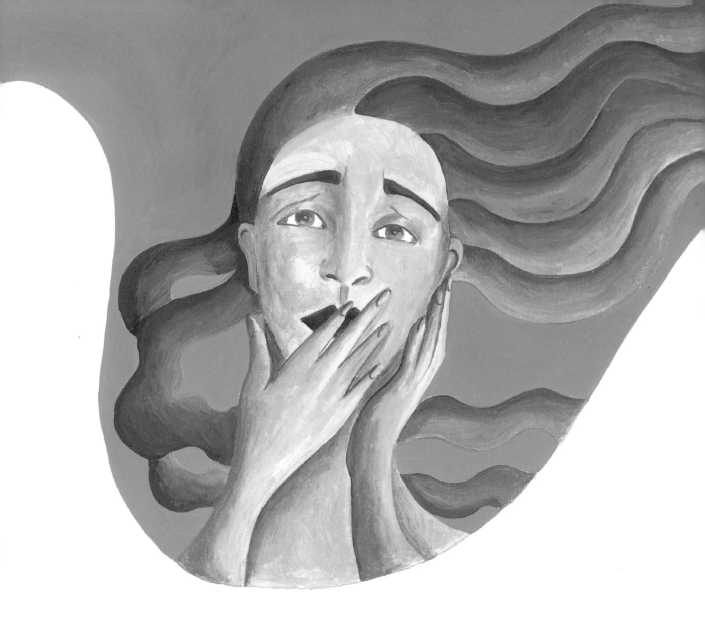

Break Out Of
"Breaking Out"

We have all suffered at some time in our lives from a "dreaded break-out". It can just be that pimple that appears prominently at the very worst time on the end of our nose, or an embarrassing itching rash that keeps coming back! Sometimes by understanding the causes, the condition can be cured; sometimes medical treatment is needed. Almost always, there is a solution. This chapter describes the most commonly experienced problems, and how to break that break-out cycle.

Acne is not just kid's stuff. It is is an all too famil-iar and a very frustrating condition. Prior to the improved treatments that have been developed during the past 15 years, acne could often cause permanent disfigurement. More than 85 percent of adolescents develop some form of acne, and nearly 95 percent of all adults suffer from acne at some time in their lives: in fact, some people acquire acne first as adults. Contrary to popular belief, acne is a disease that certain individuals do not outgrow.

The good news is that, regardless of age, acne can be treated: first, by identifying the cause and preventing the damaging factors, and second, by treatment with both shop-brought products and prescription medications.

Types of acne

Acne can range from the occasional appearance of a few isolated spots which can be a tremen-dous source of embarrassment to widespread breakouts of cysts and pustules which can even leave scars, especially on the face or back. Espe-cially when persistent and severe, acne can cause a loss of self-esteem and much needless psycho-logical distress. Acne can lead to permanent scarring if improperly treated or left untreated.

Everyone can recognize acne. Now that you understand the structure of your skin from Chap-ter 2, you will understand how acne occurs. As you learned, a sebaceous gland secretes protec-tive sebum into each hair follicle which itself is lined with dead surface cells. If dead cells accu-mulate within or on the surface of the follicle, they can combine with the sebum to cause clog-ging and distention. The normal bacteria of the skin can then multipliy within the clogged pore. Five types of blemishes can arise:

Whiteheads form when dead cells and other material inside the follicle collect and block the orifice: the opening of the skin is only a very small pore.

Blackheads are like whiteheads except that the plugging material protrudes above the open-ing of the skin surface, dilating the pore. The black coloration isn't dirt! Sebum and dead cells within the follicle oxidize, turning dark in color.

Inflammatory lesions (*papules* and *pustules*) are formed when pressure builds within the blocked follicle, and the follicle walls break under the skin. Then sebum, dead cells, and bacteria leak out into the dermis, and the skin around the pore becomes red and inflamed.

With this initial inflammation a tender, red *papule* forms on the surface of the skin. Like a balloon bursting from over-expansion, the follicle ruptures and spills its irritating contents of sebum and dead skin cells into the surrounding skin. White blood cells enter the area to attack this material, forming pus, and a *pustule* results.

When the inflammation spreads deep within the skin, a *cyst* forms. The irritating material is walled off by cells which make a fibrous capsule in order to contain the inflammation. Cysts can grow very slowly under the skin and usually require surgical treatment for removal.

Scars result when the skin tissue, damaged by acne inflammation, heals with extra, firm colla-gen, causing indentations that may be permanent. Scars often result from this healing process, but if an individual picks at the pustules, the scars can become deeper.

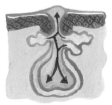

Whitehead

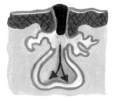

Blackhead

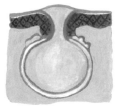

Papule

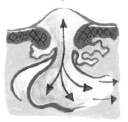

Pustule

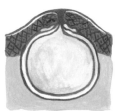

Cyst

Origins of acne

Anything that increases the sticking of cells to the skin or the secretion of sebum can cause acne. The three main influences are hormones, diet (and medications), and the products you use on your skin.

Hormones

These are those magical chemicals that are secreted by your endocrine glands to regulate your metabolism, your sexuality, your growth, your cycles, your mood and your reaction to stress. The hormones that affect your skin come primarily from your sexual organs and from your adrenal glands, the latter of which become more active when you feel either excitement or anxiety. When the adrenals are stimulated they produce more hormones.

An excess of male hormones (the level varies from individual to individual and from day to day) can lead to acne. The adrenal glands are not able to distinguish between physical fear, stress, ordinary anxiety or even great happiness, so any type of excitement, good or bad, can lead to the formation of blemishes.

Both men and women produce male androgen hormones and female estrogen hormones; however, obviously, the sexes differ in the ratio of these hormones to each other. When the relative amount of male hormones increases, as it does in certain growth spurts (particularly in teenagers), one of the results can be acne. Furthermore, just before the menstrual period in a woman, the estrogen levels are reduced and progesterone, which is chemically similar to male androgens, becomes dominant, often causing pre-menstrual acne.

A woman's body has a higher androgen to estrogen ratio during ovulation and menstruation as well as at childbirth, so again acne can flare particularly at those times. Furthermore, certain birth control pills have relatively more progesterone which can cause acne flare-ups in some individuals.

Steroids may be necessary for treating certain diseases but are often misused by athletes to build muscles. High doses can cause a very particular kind of acne with flocks of pustules which form particularly on the upper chest and back. Also, steroid creams can cause similar pustules on the treated skin .

70

Diet

It is not a myth that what you eat can affect your face! The susceptibility is quite particular for each person. Some foods are well-known culprits, such as chocolate and nuts, though not everyone who eats these gets acne. You might get acne after eating just a particular kind of nut such as peanuts or pistachios or cashews, or after eating high-fat foods such as potato chips or even stir-fried Chinese food. Very frequently dairy products can cause acne in certain people, particularly rich cheeses, ice cream, and even yogurt. If you have acne and consume a lot of dairy products, consider stopping these for a while to see if your complexion improves.

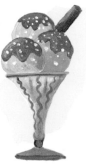

Other foods which sound healthy, such as artichokes, spinach and kale as well as seaweed and shellfish, all have a high iodide content, which can cause acne even in individuals who ordinarily would not develop this condition. Also, some soft drinks contain brominated vegetable oils that can aggravate acne.

Similarly, some medications can cause acne, particularly those that contain bromides and iodides (as many medications for asthma and colds). Lithium, used in the treatment of manic-depression, almost always causes acne when a high dose is given. Other medications that have been reported to cause acne are the sedative phenobarbital, the tuberculosis medication isoniazid, phenyltoin (used for the treatment of epilepsy), and danazole (a synthetic androgen used for the treatment of endometriosis). Even certain vitamins, particularly multi-vitamins with iodides, may provoke acne. In all of these cases, the acne will clear up if the medication or vitamin is stopped.

Environment

Finally, anything that you apply to your skin may cause so-called *acne cosmetica* or *pomade acne*. If your skin feels irritated by any particular cleanser, makeup, sunscreen, moisturizer, or even shampoo, and especially by hair treatments, it reacts by forming an extra shell of protection. How does it do this? Simply by adhering more dead cells onto the surface! It is therefore not the cosmetic *per se* that causes acne, but rather the body's protective reaction that clogs the pores.

The most frequent cause of children getting pimples around the mouth (*perioral acne*) is from bubble gum or from brushing their teeth (and the skin around their mouths!) with a fluoride toothpaste. Adults can also get fluoride acne around their mouths, often more prominently on the side on which they sleep. If you or your children have this problem, use a non-fluoride toothpaste in the evening before sleeping, and wash your face immediately after brushing.

You can even get acne from the clothes you wear. Men especially are prone to getting acne on their neck, often because their aftershave is concentrated under their collar. Wool and synthetic fabric turtlenecks can cause friction and irritation as well as increased perspiration, all exacerbating a tendency for acne.

Athletes who wear headbands or hats with

bands can get *headband acne* across their fore-head, and hikers can get *backpack acne* from sweating under their backpacks. Just changing your habits can improve your skin!

You should be particularly aware of not touching your face, especially if you have to handle prints, cleaning agents, or chemicals or even just newspapers and copy machine paper, both of which are coated with formaldehyde. Recurrent touching places the irritant onto your face, often causing either rashes or acne.

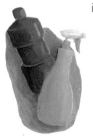

Finally, although the sun tends to dry the skin's surface and often seems to improve the complexion (although you now know otherwise), the sun itself stimulates sebum secretion and makes acne worse, even weeks after exposure. If you get pustules when you first go into the sun early in the summer, it may be your suntan oil (which you should never use, since it accelerates the sun damage to your skin) or your sunscreen. (I recommend the non-acne causing sunscreen Longévité® with SPF 25.) If you tend to develop pustules a few weeks after sun exposure, it may be because the sun has actually changed the skin lining your follicles, causing so-called *Mallorca* or *actinic acne*.

Fighting acne from outside in

Acne can very often be effectively treated by special cleansers and topically applied formulations. There are four main non-prescription acne medications which alone or in combination with prescription medications are the mainstay for

acne treatment. All of these are also available in stronger prescription form.

Salicylic acid is one of the most effective topical medications. This is a beta-hydroxy acid that is a peeling agent, because it is "keratolytic" and loosens dead surface cells that stick within pores, thereby curing clogged pores at the very onset. *Sulfur* and *resorcinol* are not only keratolytic, but also anti-bacterial. They are often mixed as flesh-tinted lotions to cover blemishes (Longévité Concealer). Sulfur is particularly effective for people with a pink or ruddy complexion.

I formulate Longévité skincare products, including a Therapeutic Cleanser with salicylic acid and sulfur. This is particularly effective in controlling acne and in smoothing the surface of the skin and making pores appear smaller. The Longévité Exfoliant immediately removes dead surface cells, which both makes the skin clearer and unclogs the pores.

The fourth highly effective, non-prescription ingredient for the treatment of acne is *benzoyl peroxide*, an anti-bacterial product available in both over-the-counter and prescription preparations. Benzoyl peroxide acts by releasing oxygen to kill bacteria and is keratolytic. Benzoyl peroxide can be purchased in gel, cream and lotion forms at the strength of 2.5%, 5% and 10% (the higher concentrations are by prescription only). Often dabbing 10% benzoyl peroxide directly onto a new spot successfully dries it out. In general, the gel forms are more effective, but can be rather drying. Benzoyl peroxide should be started at low concentrations and applied only once per day. It is important to start slowly since some people may be allergic.

If your acne does not respond to some combination of store-bought medications, you should consult a dermatologist, who may prescribe stronger formulations alone or in combination with prescription medications such as topical antibiotics or retinoic acid.

Antibiotics need not be taken orally to treat acne; they can be very effective when simply applied to the skin. Topical antibiotics exist in many forms: most frequently prescribed are clindamycin (Cleocin) and erythromycin in alcohol solutions (ATS, Eryderm, Staticin), as an ointment (Aknemycin), and on disposable pads (Erycette Pledgets) as well as in combination with benzoyl peroxide (Benzamycin Gel). The alcohol solutions can be drying, so they should be applied at least 15 or 20 minutes after washing your face. Naturally, if you experience any burning, stinging, itching or redness after using any of these medications you should discontinue them straightaway and tell your doctor, who will recommend an alternative.

The prescription medication which is perhaps the most effective anti-acne medication available is retinoic acid or Retin A, the natural form of vitamin A found in the skin. Since the late 1960s retinoic acid has been used as a medication for treating acne. Its major action is keratolytic, so that cells within the blocked pores no longer stick to the skin surface.

The problem with retinoic acid is that it can be irritating, causing dry, red flaky skin, especially when first used. Some people cannot use retinoic acid, even at a low concentration. Retinoic acid also increases the skin's sensitivity to the sun and to any other products applied to the skin, such as perfumes and cosmetics.

Retin A is a very powerful prescription drug. It is available in six forms. You need apply only a tiny amount of Retin A to the acne-prone areas of your skin at night about 10 minutes after washing your face. The great news is that Retin A is also effective in correcting tiny wrinkles and dark spots caused by exposure to the sun.

An exciting new medication which has been available in Europe since 1989 but is not yet widely used in the United States is *azeleic acid*, a natural acid found in cereal grains. It acts differently from other medications, altering the structure of the outer skin cells so that they are less adherent. It also directly kills bacteria and inhibits melanin formation, thereby preventing and treating darkened scars from acne and mottled pigmentation from sun damage. Azeleic acid may prove to be even better than retinoic acid, with less dryness and sensitization.

Fighting acne from inside out

If the acne is so severe that it cannot be effectively prevented or treated using topical medications, oral medications are often necessary. These are reserved for the tougher, more resistant cases of acne.

The most commonly used oral medications are *antibiotics,* the most widely prescribed of which is tetracycline. Tetracycline not only kills the

great skin for life

bacteria but also reduces sebum secretion. It must be taken on an empty stomach (one hour before or two hours after a meal). Tetracycline binds to calcium, so it is not absorbed if taken with dairy products. Tetracycline should not be taken by children under ten or by pregnant women or women who are breastfeeding, since it can stain a child's developing teeth.

Other effective antibiotics are minocycline, erythromycin and doxycycline. The effectiveness of each particular antibiotic is highly individual. Certain antibiotics work extremely well on some people, but not on others. Some people experience slight nausea when an antibiotic is taken in the morning before eating. Other frequent side-effects are diarrhea and vaginal yeast infections (Candida, monilia).

The type of antibiotic used and the dose must be determined under your doctor's care.

Finally, there is a "magic medicine" for acne called *13-cis-retinoic acid* or *Accutane*, a synthetic derivative of vitamin A. This is a very strong oral medication which is taken once or twice a day for four months, after which acne is usually cured. Before beginning this medication, your blood must be checked to be certain that the liver metabolizes normally. Throughout the course of medication, monthly blood tests of cholesterol and triglyceride are necessary, since any changes in triglyceride might alter the dose.

Everyone taking Accutane has some feeling of dryness of the lips and often skin sensitivity and dryness of the eyes and nose. Sometimes even individuals experience nose bleeds or sore gums because of the dry mucosal membranes. If these symptoms are uncomfortable, often the dose of

the medication will be decreased. The most major potential problem with Accutane is that it would cause birth defects if ever taken by a pregnant woman. Women must not become pregnant while taking Accutane. Very strict birth control must be used when on Accutane, and pregnancy itself is not safe until two months after the course of the medication is completed.

What your dermatologist can do

Besides determining the exact cause of your acne and prescribing the correct medications, your dermatologist can very quickly treat blackheads, new spots and cysts. Usually the dermatologist accomplishes this by treating the affected area with a fine scalpel blade and expressing the contents. If you have a deep cyst, the dermatologist can drain it or inject medication. The sooner the inflammation is under control, the less likely there is to be any permanent scarring.

Finally, there are treatments for acne scarring. Most common are injections of collagen directly into the scar. Often each scar requires more than one treatment but after several treatments the correction is permanent. In some cases of extensive scarring, the surgical procedures of dermabrasion or the more modern laser abrasion can be effective. These procedures are described in detail in Chapter 10. Fortunately with the medications now available, major scarring can usually be prevented.

Eczema

The word *eczema* is derived from a Greek word meaning "to boil out", a description of the family of itchy skin conditions which begin with

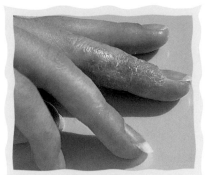

Eczema of the hands not only itches but can also be very painful.

redness and swelling, often followed by blisters and oozing, then scaling, and finally thick, leathery, frequently painfully cracked skin. Several categories of eczema exist, the most common of which are atopic dermatitis, hand dermatitis, and nummular dermatitis.

Atopic dermatitis is a common condition all over the world, affecting about three percent of the American population. It runs in families whose members also suffer from other allergies such as hay fever and asthma. Atopic dermatitis usually first appears in infancy with redness and chapping on the baby's cheeks and scalp. The infant suffers intolerable itching and cries constantly. A consolation is that half of these babies recover before they are two.

If the atopy continues, the dermatitis affects the back of the arms and the front of the legs, then subsequently shifts to the skin in the folds of the elbows, knees, and neck. The affected skin becomes dry and scaly from the constant scratching. Most patients recover before age 25.

Atopic dermatitis can be partially alleviated by avoiding irritants in the environment. Any clothing worn close to the skin should be soft cotton, silk or nylon – wool should never be worn. All new clothing should be washed before wearing. Feather pillows and wool blankets should not be used, and fuzzy or woollen toys must be avoided with children. If kept indoors, dogs, cats and birds can worsen atopic dermatitis. The child should be protected from dust as well as from irritating household cleansers, detergents, greases, oils, and harsh soaps. Humidifiers in winter protect against dry heat, and air conditioners in summer can alleviate sweating. Certain foods can provoke flareups: milk, eggs, fish, wheat, peanuts, chocolate, and citrus fruits.

Individuals with atopic dermatitis are very susceptible to infections such as the herpes virus. They are also likely to develop severe reactions to injections of penicillin and certain other drugs. A child should not be vaccinated when experiencing atopic dermatitis.

Fortunately, there are effective treatments which can alleviate the itching. Just bathing less frequently helps: children do not need to be washed daily! The application of topical steroid creams once or twice each day with emollients in between can also stop the inflammation-itch cycle. Sometimes oral antihistamines are needed.

Hand dermatitis in an adult might be the only remnant of childhood atopic dermatitis. This is a chronic dryness, itching, and painful fissuring of the skin on the hands that can lead to swelling and infection. It is usually a reaction to common irritants such as soap, detergents, and solvents, common in housewives ("dishpan hands"), food handlers, bartenders, nurses and dentists.

Hand eczemas of entirely different causes may closely resemble each other. *Allergic contact dermatitis* may be caused by contact with one specific chemical, but everyday hand contacts are so numerous that identification can be difficult. The pattern of the rash and patch tests determine the cause. *Psoriasis* on the hands is usually accompanied by psoriasis on the body and a family history of the disease. *Dyshidrotic hand eczema* is characterized by tiny, deep, itchy blisters, which appear suddenly on the sides of the fingers and palms, especially often in people who tend to perspire excessively on the palms and soles of the feet. *Fungal infections* may be diagnosed by doing a culture or looking for organisms in the microscope. *ID reactions* are allergic rashes on the hands associated with an infection elsewhere on the body (usually on the feet).

The precise cause of the hand dermatitis must be identified, often requiring a visit to your dermatologist. It is always advisable to avoid touching all irritants. Rings should be removed when washing the hands; mild soaps must be used and the hands should be dried thoroughly and an emollient applied afterwards. Whenever any irritant is encountered (including even newsprint), white cotton gloves should be worn. If solvents or household cleansers and detergents are used, rubber gloves should be worn over the cotton gloves. Severe cases should be treated medically, usually with topical steroids or tar preparations.

Nummular dermatitis is characterized by coin-shaped, itchy, dry patches that are scattered over the body or arms and legs. These occur most frequently in older people. This irritation may relate to a previous atopic dermatitis, a reaction to irritants, or just a reaction to dry environments

and winter weather. Usually the condition improves in the summer but worsens under emotional stress. As with hand dermatitis, treatment involves eliminating contact with irritants and application of topical steroids. Keeping the skin well-moisturized is a must.

Allergic contact dermatitis

Almost everything can cause an allergy in someone, somewhere! The medical literature is full of reports of strange skin allergies: clarinet players with lip blisters from an allergy to the bamboo reed; drivers with allergic reactions to steering wheels; chefs with allergies to pineapple juice, corn and other moist foods.

An *allergic* contact dermatitis is a specific sensitivity in a person with a genetic predisposition. In contrast an *irritant* contact dermatitis occurs in everyone who touches the irritating substance (as described previously), though some people are more sensitive than others, reacting to lower concentrations or fewer contacts. To suffer an allergic reaction, that person must already have been exposed to the substance. The skin irritation appears after a second or third (or even a one-thousandth) contact only on the specific area which touched the allergen.

Gardeners and flower arrangers beware! The most common allergic contact dermatitis results from contact with plants, especially poison ivy in the United States or poison sumac in Europe (hence the saying: Leaflets three, let it be). Exposure happens by inadvertently brushing against the leaves and then depositing the plant's oil (oleoresin) on the skin. A characteristic red, swollen, blistering, itchy skin irritation develops 12 to 48 hours later. Lovely flowers can also cause this uncomfortable and sometimes frightening reaction, including chrysanthemum and dahlias when injured, the "hairs" of orchids and primroses, and tulip bulbs.

A common misconception is that the blister fluid on the skin is contagious. This is not true! The blistering appears to evolve with more blisters appearing over several days because initially the plant oil was deposited in varying concentrations. The earliest blisters are areas exposed to high concentrations of the oil; later blisters had less concentrated contact. If you realize you have touched a plant allergen, wash the area thoroughly (including under your fingernails!) within 20 minutes of contact to prevent the rash. Remember to wash everything that was in contact with the plant, because unless completely removed, the oil can remain active for years. The burning of many plants causes the oil to vaporize, thereby contacting all exposed skin and often causing very severe allergic dermatitis.

Another very frequent cause of allergic dermatitis is nickel, a frustrating problem since nickel is everywhere! Necklaces, earrings, rings, bracelets, costume jewelry, hairpins, belt buckles, watch bands, zippers (zips), scissors, door handles, pens, knitting needles, screws in orthopaedic implants, coins – all contain nickel! You can test for nickel by purchasing a kit containing dimethylglyoxine. If you are allergic, you can cover these commonly used objects and even jewelry with cellophane wrap or with clear nail varnish. Stainless steel or gold jewelry can be worn. Be sure that any cooking utensils are made of stainless steel, enamel, or are coated.

Other common causes of contact allergy are chromatin (in different materials such as cement, photographic processes, metals, dyes, detergents, rubber, leather, and cosmetic ingredients.

Major causes of allergic contact dermatitis

AREA	CAUSE
Scalp	Shampoo, hair dyes
Ears	Metal earrings, eye glasses
Eyelids	Nail polish, formaldehyde from paper or fabric (both transferred by touching), eye shadow, mascara, contact lens solution
Face	Airborne allergens (burning leaves, ragweed), makeup sunscreens, medications (most commonly benzoyl peroxide), after-shave, perfumes
Neck	Necklaces, perfumes, after-shave lotions, hair dyes
Body	Topical medications, sunscreens, plants, clothing, undergarments (especially elastic bands), metal belt, buckles, adhesive bandages
Underarms	Deodorants, clothing, detergent or bleach (from clothing)
Arms / hands	Watches and watchbands, soaps, detergents and foods
Genitals	Plants (transferred by hand), rubber condoms
Lower legs	Topical medications, dye or detergent in socks
Feet	Shoes (rubber or leather)

Obviously the treatment is to avoid the allergens! You and your dermatologist must work together as detectives to discover the precise cause. Sometimes a patch test (applying all possible culprits to the skin for two days) is necessary. Patch testing is important in allergies to cosmetics, since the precise component can be identified and avoided. Meanwhile, the itchy rash can be treated with topical steroids.

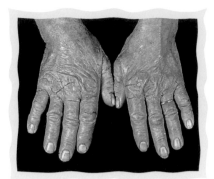

A blistering contact dematitis can simply come from touching or handling the wrong thing.

Hives

These localized swellings (urticaria or wheals) of the skin or mucous membranes are usually very itchy. They can occur suddenly, last a few hours and then disappear, leaving no trace. No single hive lasts more than 36 hours. By circling the irregular, red swelling with a pen, you will see that it fades, even as new ones form. Each hive can be as small as a pea to larger than 30 cm (12in). When a hive forms near the eyes, lips, or genitals, there can be a frightening swelling called *angioedema* which lasts 12–24 hours (if the throat swells, seek urgent medical attention).

Hives are caused by the release of the natural chemical histamine from mast cells which lie along blood vessels in the skin. Histamine release can be triggered directly by certain natural chemicals in certain foods (such as strawberries and shellfish), drugs (especially aspirin and other salicyclates), or food preservatives such as tartrazine (a yellow dye often found in canned vegetables) or monosodium glutamate (MSG, frequently in Chinese food). Histamine release can also be caused by an allergy to a food or a topically applied cream or, less frequently, by a physical allergy to cold, heat, or even just pressure.

About one in every five people will have hives sometime in their lives. In most cases, a person suffers only one or two episodes which last less than six weeks. This is *acute urticaria*, usually caused by foods, drugs, an insect bite or an infection such as chicken pox, viral respiratory infections, mononucleosis, intestinal parasites, serum hepatitis, and rheumatic fever. People who have these brief attacks can usually be their own

Common hand irritants

Soap	Fruits
Detergents	*(especially citrus)*
Cleansers	Vegetables
Bleaches	*(especially garlic, okra,*
Hair preparations	*onions, potatoes)*
(e.g. shampoos,	Paper, newsprint
colorings and	Raw meats
conditioners, etc.)	Laquers
Urine in diaper	Floor, furniture, or
(nappy)	car polishes
Wool	Gasoline, lighter fluid
Alcohol	Paints, paint thinners

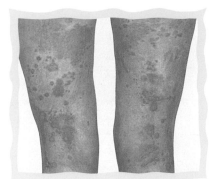

Hives can come and go; the causes are many and varied.

detectives in determining the cause by simply keeping a careful "diet diary" of everything that enters their mouths from foods, medications and vitamins to mouthwash, toothpaste and chewing gum, and then listing when the hives occur.

Hives usually appear ten minutes to eight hours after eating the offending food. A more tedious method to investigate food allergies is an elimination diet. First eliminate what you think is the culprit. If you still get hives, eat a restricted diet consisting of only four unseasoned, low-allergy foods: lamb, rice, apples and decaffeinated tea for one week. If the hives disappear, new foods can be introduced one at a time to pinpoint the culprit. If hives continue, you must eliminate even those foods one by one to detect the cause, or perhaps food is not actually the problem.

The most common medications that often cause hives are aspirin, codeine, penicillin, and sulfa drugs. Penicillin may also be found in blue and Roquefort cheeses and any dairy product. Almost every medication has been a cause of urticaria in some person somewhere. The coating of pills or capsules can also bring about hives.

Some people develop hives minutes after exposure to sun; others suffer from *heat* or *cold* *urticaria*, which can occur with mild temperature changes, as in taking a hot shower or plunging into a tepid swimming pool on a hot day. Urticaria may be accompanied by wheezing, flushing, and fainting if exposure is prolonged.

People with hives demonstrate *dermographism* or "skin writing", so that even stroking the skin causes a wheal lasting 30 minutes to several hours. Dermographism is a minor inconvenience, but rarely a person with severe *pressure urticaria* is unable to grasp a steering wheel or tennis racket without itching and swelling.

Bouts of urticaria lasting more than six weeks are classified as *chronic urticaria*. People who have a personal or family history of asthma, hay fever, or migraine headaches seem more susceptible to stubborn chronic hives. Although the exact cause is sometimes never ascertained, it is important to do a thorough medical examination to check for infection, autoimmune disease, or hidden malignancy. Eighty percent of cases resolve spontaneously within one year.

The best treatment for hives is to discover and eliminate the cause. Meanwhile, oral antihistamines can be given for relief.

Foods causing attacks of hives

Shellfish	Cheese	Citrus fruits
Beef	Milk	Strawberries
Pork	Chocolate	Corn
Eggs	Sweeteners	Tomatoes
Nuts		Wheat
Seasonings		
(ketchup, mayonnaise, mustard, spices)		

The Basics of Skin "Care"

OK...where do we stand? Chapter 2 taught us something of the structure of skin. In Chapter 3, you completed a detailed personal analysis of your skin. In Chapters 4 and 5 you learned that your outdoor and indoor environments influence your skin. You examined your body for lumps and bumps in Chapter 6, and identified some special skin problems in Chapter 7. Now it's time to learn how you can take advantage of advances in medical and scientific research to really "care" for your skin.

This chapter shares with you my experience and knowledge about the essentials of skincare: cleansing, exfoliating, shaving, moisturizing and treating particular problems. The most important thing to remember as you read is that skincare is very individual, tailored to your own needs and your own lifestyle.

You will learn a number of different methods for each aspect of skincare, as well as how to evaluate the skincare products that you should use. It's up to you to use your good taste, your experience, and your common sense in taking care of yourself.

All of us have "combination" skin, meaning that different parts of our skin require different care. Moreover, as you learned from your personal analysis, everybody's skin changes with age, the seasons, the climate, the environment, stress, and lifestyle: your skincare routine can and should also adapt to all of these variables. You will learn how to accommodate your skincare to your ever-evolving life!

Excellent skincare isn't difficult; it isn't time consuming; it isn't expensive. Just minutes each day of *correct* care can truly change how you look. You owe it to yourself to keep your skin – the very beautiful wrapping with which we were born – in good shape. No matter what your particular difficulty, it can be helped, and usually in a relatively short time. Remember, the whole skin surface renews itself every 30 days!

The short time necessary to dedicate to your skincare are both a necessity and a wonderful luxury. With a little attention to proper skincare, you will give yourself the gift of beauty through youthful, healthy, radiant skin.

Cleansing for Great Skin

Proper cleansing can be the *most important* part of your skincare routine! Not only is it absolutely necessary to get your face *clean* without irritating your skin (often a delicate balance), but you can also *treat* your skin by the way you wash and the soap or cleanser you use. Your bath or shower can be your best friend, your greatest indulgence and your most important key to excellent health and a great, young appearance.

Getting the product right!

As you learned in Chapter 2, your skin is by nature slightly acidic (with a pH of about 5.5). Until recently, most soaps and cleansers were the opposite – slightly alkaline. The result was dry skin! With advances in cosmetic chemistry, no longer do you have to choose from only harsh, alkaline products. With space age technology, you can test for possible irritants in cleansing products and measure their effectiveness with good accuracy. Although your grandmothers or mother cautioned you never to use soap on your face, that advice is no longer up-to-date. Indeed, with the excellent cleansing products that now exist, it is foolish not to benefit!

Yes, but there's a problem: how to choose. The number of product choices is mind-boggling! To begin to help you decide what cleanser you should choose – soap, liquid cleanser, cream or lotion – for your own skin, let's look at the basics.

Choosing a soap

All soaps are combinations of a fat source which lifts away oil and grease – either tallow (from the solid fats of cattle and sheep) or an oil (coconut, palm, peanut, to name a few) – and a salt-like alkaline compound which allows the soap-dirt mixture to dissolve in water for removal.

A *mild* or *gentle soap* is not all soap; it contains a lot of moisturizing cream. *Super-fatted soaps* have relatively more fat; they are less alkaline and therefore milder, but they rinse off less effectively. *Transparent soaps* are made with glycerin and alcohol, and are best for oily skin. *French-milled soaps* are merely denser than other soaps; they are pressed so they contain less moisture and less air. Milled soaps last longer and lather well; they sink in the tub! In contrast, *floating soaps* have extra air so they disappear rapidly. *Deodorant soaps* contain antibacterial agents which kill the bacteria that cause body odor.

There are many *specialty soaps* (some sound good enough to eat!): Castile soap with olive oil; cocoa butter, nut, or fruit oil soaps; oatmeal soap. Soaps containing aloe vera or vitamin E sound good, but they actually give no special benefit to the skin since their potentially helpful ingredients are not in contact with the skin for long enough to be absorbed, and are not in a form that is useful on the skin.

Detergents and *synthetic soaps* were developed during the Second World War. With the wartime shortage of fats and oils, the fats in soaps were replaced with synthetic or natural hydrocarbons. Many detergents exist; they're not all for dishes and clothes! There are mild synthetic cleansing agents. Their advantage is that they make pleasant soapy suds, even in mineral-rich hard water; and they leave no grimy ring around the bathtub.

Liquid facial and *body cleansers* or "cleansing solutions" contain the same kinds of ingredients as soap; they are liquid because there is more water in the formulation, but the concentration of active ingredients is similar. (The advantage is that there is no messy bar dissolving in a soap dish.) Further in this chapter, I use the words cleanser and soap interchangeably. Your own choice of product will depend upon your skin type, your preference and your personal evaluation of each product.

Cleansing lotions

Cleansing lotions and creams are mostly variants of the Roman physician Galen's cold cream. They contain a combination of mineral or synthetic oil and wax or petrolatum (or vaseline) which melts on contact with warm skin to dissolve oils and loosen grime. Lotions are "cold" since the water or menthol in the formula evaporate, cooling the skin – the more water, the colder they are. Some cleansing lotions were formulated especially to wipe off greasy or waterproof makeup (particularly mascara). Other lotions are used like soaps and rinsed off with water, rather than wiped off. I recommend that after using a cleansing cream or lotion (unless you are only touching up a makeup smudge), you always wash with a soap or cleanser and then rinse.

The right cleanser

So which cleanser should you choose? As mentioned before, *everyone* has combination skin. Almost everyone, therefore, would benefit from using a different cleanser in the oily section of the face – the forehead, nose and chin or "T-zone" – than for the drier cheeks and neck, and perhaps still another cleansing product for the body. If your face is especially oily in the morning, after exercise, or after a stressful day at work, use an anti-oil cleanser at that time, with ingredients such as sulfur, salicylic acid, or benzoyl peroxide.

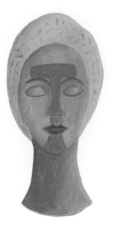

The face is most oily in the "T-zone of the fore-head, nose and chin.

Your skin may change seasonally or in different environments. It might be drier in the winter or the summer (if you foolishly went into the sun) or after a long flight. Everyone should always have at least two cleansers – one for the treatment of oily areas and a milder cleanser for dryness. Although this may sound unnecessarily complicated, it is actually quite simple and the benefits are enormous.

You must be careful to use milder cleansers on your face and hands (which you probably wash more frequently) than on your body. A medical, antibacterial cleanser may be recommended to you by your dermatologist (even for your face) if you have acne. Always avoid using "popular" deodorant cleansers and highly perfumed cleansers on your face, especially if you have particularly dry or sensitive skin. The deodorants and perfumes in these products may act as irritants and they may also be photosensitizing.

Washing can be fun!

The way you wash your skin is as important as the cleansing agent you choose! Washing incorrectly can be truly detrimental to your skin. The chart on the following page contains a few simple facts about how to wash your face. Below you will find some important and useful tips to follow when bathing or showering.

Ten bathing tips

In the busy lives we lead today, people often shower rapidly. We can benefit greatly, however, from the luxury of relaxing in a bath. This time can be a real beauty treatment – for your face, your body, and your soul! To get the most out of your bath or shower and to appreciate these relaxing minutes of your day, here are some suggestions:

1   The ideal temperature for showering or relaxing in your bath without becoming drowsy is about 95°F (35°C). The steam is very good to open the pores of your face for a thorough cleaning. (It's also therapeutic if you have a cold with congestion.) If you have a tendency to develop spider veins on your legs, avoid very hot baths and jacuzzis, and when you are in a warm bath, lie so that your body is submerged but your hips are raised out of the water. If you have a tendency to facial redness or flushing, try lowering the temperature of the bath a bit.

2   As you first lie in the tub or step into the shower, luxuriating in the warmth, you could do a few isometric exercises to stimulate your muscles. Some of the Pressometrics from my previous book *Thin Thighs For Life* are great! Do the Flapper and the Power Palm Press five

times each when you get in; then squeeze your buttocks and abdominal muscles into the Hip Hugger and repeat five times. Finally, with your legs straight, press your knees together, feeling the contraction of your inner thighs in each Kneecap Kiss. Do five repetitions. Your body will be more streamlined and your posture improved in less than two minutes!

3   For the ultimate in relaxation, deep-breathing can be wonderful. Inhale deeply through your nose to a count of four, expanding your chest and your abdomen as you lower your diaphragm. Hold your breath for a count of eight, exhale slowly through your mouth for a count of 12. Repeat five times.

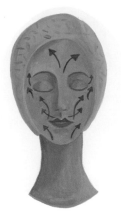

Treat your wrinkles while you are washing: rub up and rub out.

4   Now lie back and close your eyes. Relax all your muscles, from the tips of your fingers to the tips of your toes; relax your spine, your legs, your arms, your neck and your facial muscles.

5   It is better not to soak or shower for more than 30 minutes. The first 15 minutes are certainly very good for your skin as the outer layer of dead skin cells takes in water - the only true skin moisturization. But with longer sessions, your fingers and toes can become puffy and rigged.

6   If you use bubblebath, be sure to rinse in a shower before drying. It is not good for your skin to have a coating of residual soap.

7   As good as it might feel, I do not recommend bath oil – first because of the very real danger

Cleansing for a Beautiful Face: Nine Tips

1   Wash your hands thoroughly before you wash your face.

2   Wash with warm, not hot, water, especially if your face often flushes. Not only can hot water actually burn you, but it worsens the natural tendency to develop extra blood vessels on your face, giving an unattractive, ruddy complexion.

3   Wash your face and neck with upward, outward motions. On your face, always rub perpendicular to the direction of those wrinkles that you could develop later. On the forehead, cheeks, chin and neck, rub up and out; above your upper lip and under your eyes, the strokes should be first horizontal, then upward at the edges.

4   Rinse, rinse, rinse! It's very important to remove all cleanser from your skin. To test how well your cleanser rinses in the particular water you use, add some soap or cleanser to a clear glass of water, leave for a few minutes, then rinse. If there's a layer coating the glass, this may be a clue that you should rinse extra-carefully. Be aware that your cleanser will not rinse off as well if you travel to an area with mineral-rich, "hard" water.

5   Be sure not to get cleanser in your eyes, especially if you use a product with abrasive grains. If any does get into your eyes, wash thoroughly by cupping you hand and rinsing your eye with water.

6   Unless there is a particular problem with the water source (as might be encountered in a less developed country) you need not wash with special drinking water!

7   Polishing touches: some people prefer to wash with their fingertips, some with a delicate facial brush, a sponge or exfoliating pad (which will be discussed in the following section). This is a matter of personal taste and preference. Just be certain that whatever you use is clean.

8   Don't overwash. Unless you're exercising frequently and strenuously or you are in a sooty environment, it is unlikely that you ever need to wash your face more than four times a day. Everyone should wash in the morning, after exercising, in the evening after work (especially if you have applied makeup), and before bed. If your skin is oily despite frequent washing, you should used a different cleanser, an astringent, or a medication from your dermatologist.

9   Apply sunscreen, moisturizer, or other treatment creams or lotions immediately after towel-drying your face in order to seal in the essential water.

that you can slip in the tub, and second because it tends to float on the water surface and can coat your skin, preventing the real moisturization by the water. If you absolutely adore your bath oil, it is better to apply it to your damp body with a washcloth or bath-mitt after you bathe.

8 Some herbs are therapeutic. You can make a bath sachet with a 6in (15cm) square of cheese cloth; fill with ½ cup of herbs or tea, knot on top, and tie it under the faucet (taps) so that it is submerged when the bath is full.

- For scent, use bay leaves, cinnamon bark, jasmine tea, or orange peel.
- For circulation, use ginger.
- For sensitive skin, use chamomile.
- For itchy skin, sprinkle finely ground oatmeal powder into the bath.

9 After soaking, wash! Apply your cleanser to your washcloth, bathsponge, brush, polishing pad, or loofah. Rub your body with long, smooth strokes, working from the extremities inward toward your body, massaging always toward your heart. Use an exfoliant cream or a pumice stone on any extra-tough skin you might have on your soles, knees, or elbows. Rinse thoroughly. Take a quick shower after a bath to remove any residual soap.

10 Immediately after towel-drying, always be sure to apply a moisturizer to any specially dry areas of skin; particularly your feet, lower legs, and elbows might benefit. If you have cellulite on your thighs, upper arms, or love handles, now is the time to massage those areas with an anti-cellulite product, as you learned in *Thin Thighs for Life*.

The importance of exfoliation

I am devoting a special section to exfoliation because I consider this to be one of the most beneficial of skincare treatments. Why? Because so many of our skin's problems can be prevented by removing dead surface cells. Dry skin is simply the accumulation of dead skin on our skin's surface. Youthful skin, in contrast, has signifi-cantly fewer layers of dead cells than older skin. Exfoliation smoothes wrinkles and rough skin; and pimples do not form if the pores don't have dead skin debris clogging them.

The method

Exfoliation can be chemical or mechanical. The alpha- and beta-hydroxy acids and retinoic acid (described in Chapter 9) are chemical exfoliants: they unglue dead surface cells. Other exfoliants are mechanical – cleansing grains, waxy creams that adhere to the surface cells, and slightly abra-sive polishing pads, brushes, or loofahs.

When using exfoliants, don't rub too vigorously on delicate areas such as under your eyes. If you have delicate, thin skin and a tendency to develop blood vessels on your face, use a mild product and be gentle. Do not use abrasive exfoliants if you have severe acne (so you don't spread the problem as you rub!) On your face, always rub up and out, against the direction of wrinkles.

On your body, always rub towards your heart. If you have many facial wrinkles, very dry skin on your legs, and/or dry, rough skin (*keratosis pilaris*) on your upper arms or thighs, you should use an abrasive pad with a medicated cleanser on those areas. A vigorous sanding with a pumice stone helps very dry skin on the soles, elbows and knees.

A close shave

More than three out of four women shave their underarms, bikini area, and/or legs to remove excess hair, and almost all men shave their beard. The secret of a good shave is closeness with comfort. An understanding of hair growth and a proper shaving technique are important. As a dermatologist, I often see shaving-related problems such as irritation or *pseudofolliculitus* (pimples).

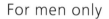

For men only

Since Alexander the Great first shaved to make it more difficult for his enemies to decapitate him without the leverage of grabbing his beard (another good reason for shaving!), the average man spends approximately 3,350 hours (over 200 16-hour days) of his lifetime removing a total of 27ft (8.4m) of hair weighing over 4lb (1.8kg) from his face. Although this might seem a time-consuming bother, men are quite lucky to have facial hair. Their beard protects their skin, so men have fewer wrinkles. Also, shaving is a great form of exfoliation, helping to smooth the skin's surface.

Most men experience their most rapid beard growth at the age of about 30. Beard growth varies with the time of day – more rapid during the day than at night. Beard growth is unaffected by shaving or external manipulation.

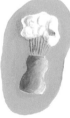

Shaving essentials

Believe it or not, beard hair, bikini line hair, and women's leg hair have about the same hardness as copper wire of the same thickness! Fortu-nately, hair doesn't stay tough, since exposure to warm water for two to four minutes causes the hair to expand 34 percent in volume, making it softer and easier to cut. (The force required to cut softened hair is reduced by nearly 70 percent.) If beard hair is not properly softened, even a sharp razor blade can be damaged in the first few strokes, and the rest of the shave is uncomfortable and damaging to the skin. It is essential, therefore, to first wash the area to be shaved with warm, soapy water and to apply shaving cream three minutes before shaving to properly soften and moisten the beard. The shaving cream provides a protective blanket to prevent evapora-tion of water, keeping the hairs soft during the shave and increasing lubricancy of the skin's surface so the blade glides smoothly, without irri-tation. Viscous lotion-like shaving creams provide better moisturization than frothy aerosol foams (which tend to dry more rapidly). Anyone who develops little pustules over shaved areas should use a medicated shaving cream containing, for example, benzoyl peroxide.

For minimal irritation, shaving should be done with the fewest possi-ble light, gentle strokes in the direction of hair growth (though shaving against the growth sometimes gives a closer shave). Women should shave their legs before their bikini area, and men should shave the whiskers on their upper lips and chins last, to assure that these coarser hairs are given maximum time to soften.

A good cutting edge is important. Razors give a closer shave; electric shavers cause less irritation. (To assure a close and safe shave with an electric razor, the skin can be prepared with cream as described above, and then rinsed off prior to shaving.) A great deal of research has been done to design "the perfect razor". The optimal angle of the blade to the skin is 28 to 30 degrees. Double-bladed razors give a closer shave. When using any razor, rinse and shake off excess water rather than wiping the blade in order to preserve the sharpness.

After-shave products

Designed to minimize "razor burn", after-shaves are usually fragranced colognes that contain cooling menthol. I recommend the least scented after-shaves because fragrances can be irritating. After-shaves based on witch-hazel instead of alcohol are less irritating to the skin. Men should apply sunscreen after shaving, since their exfoliated skin is very susceptible to sun damage. Women should not apply a deodorant or antiperspirant directly after shaving under their arms. Non-alcoholic creams or dusting powders can be soothing, especially in the bikini area.

Unwanted hair

As if women don't have enough worries, many still have to contend with unwanted facial hair. The genetic tendency to downy hair on the cheeks has been admired by many poets and novelists. Usually this soft, fine hair decreases by the age of 30. Women are dismayed, in contrast, by the appearance of thick, dark hairs on the cheeks or chin (stimulated after menopause by

the adrenal androgens no longer balanced by higher levels of ovarian estrogens). To avoid the unnecessary irritation, women should not shave hair on their faces; I recommend simply tweezing these random, unwanted hairs. Regrowth takes around two to four weeks, and repeated tweezing can sometimes damage the follicle sufficiently to thin the hair.

Women with many facial hairs or who prefer not to shave their legs or bikini area, can use one of three alternative methods:

1 *Depilatories* chemically dissolve hair. Because the outer layer of the skin is composed of a keratin protein similar to that of hair, however, depilatories are also quite irritating to the skin. Often they can be tolerated for several uses, but with time they very frequently cause allergic reactions. I suggest that you first test a small area of skin and wait 24 hours to see if there is any irritation before continuing. Follow the instructions carefully. On the face, use only a facial depilatory, and be sure to remove the depilatory within the time recommended on the packet.

2 *Waxing* pulls the hair out from the root, just as tweezing does, but unfortunately the hairs must be fairly long for optimal results, and the process is actually quite painful. Because waxing frequently causes ingrown hairs, be sure to use the exfoliating techniques described above in the area to be waxed prior to the procedure. If you wax yourself, always apply a little dusting powder prior to waxing as well as after. Be sure that the wax is not too hot. (Test the temperature of the wax

with a small amount on your inner wrist.) The wax should always be pulled against the direction of hair growth.

3 *Electrolysis,* properly performed, can permanently remove unwanted hairs. This is a painful technique, but fortunately a new anesthetic cream (Emla) can be prescribed by your doctor. It is critical to find a competent technician, since poorly performed electrolysis frequently leaves temporary dark spots or scars, and the hairs might regrow despite the pain suffered in the process.

Moisturizing your skin

Everyone suffers at some time from dry skin. When your skin is dry, you reach for a moisturizer. But effective moisturizing involves more than just day cream or lotion.

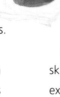

When doctors look at dry skin under a microscope, they see that it is actually an accumulation of dead cells adhering to the skin's surface. These cells are made of the protein, keratin, which can absorb water, changing from dry, tile-like flakes to smooth, plump cells. Natural, moist, supple skin depends upon the complex interaction of these surface cells with the environment, with water, with your body's secretions, or with moisturizers you apply.

Moisturizing your skin is a four-step process, as follows: 1) prevention of excess dryness as best you can by proper cleansing and avoiding harsh environments; 2) removing the excess dry dead surface cells by exfoliation; 3) bringing water to the skin's surface; and 4) preventing that water from evaporating. The last two steps can be achieved by using a good quality moisturizer!

The body has two kinds of natural moisturizer:
• Natural moisturizing factors (NMFs), which attract and bind water.
• Lipids secreted by the sebaceous glands, which seal in that water.

NMFs include amino acids; urea; phospholipids; creatinine; lactic, glycolic, and uric acids, to name a few. Although harsh washing can temporally deplete the skin of its NMFs and natural lipids, these are normally replenished within hours. More important, in dry environments (especially under 40 percent humidity), any water on the surface of our warm skin evaporates, drying the surface. Skin surface lipids are essential, to seal in the moisture.

Types of moisturizer

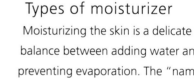

Moisturizing the skin is a delicate balance between adding water and preventing evaporation. The "name of the game" is to decrease "transepidermal water loss" (TEWL). This means getting the water to the surface cells and then keeping it there!

Humectants (like NMFs) attract water to the skin's surface. Unless environmental humidity exceeds 70 percent, the water on your skin's surface comes from the deeper layers of your epidermis and from your dermis. If the body is warmer than the surrounding environment, that surface water evaporates resulting in increased water loss. After several hours of this evaporation, the skin is even drier then before and the humectant must be reapplied (much to the joy of the cosmetic companies who sell you the product).

A humectant alone, therefore, is not enough; a good moisturizer must have something to keep the moisture on the skin's surface from evaporating – an occlusive ingredient.

Examples of humectants are glycerine, honey, propyline glycol (which can cause occasional allergic reaction), butylene glycol, sorbitol, gelatin, lecithin, pyrrolidone carboxylic acid (PCA), and hyaluronic acid. Collagen, elastin, and DNA serve very important functions within our bodies, but when applied to the surface of the skin they are simply expensive humectants. Their molecules are too large to be absorbed through the skin, and they cannot possibly function from the skin's surface in building skin structure or stimulating reproduction of cells, despite what advertisements might suggest. Neither do I recommend placental extract which serves as a surface humectant, but nothing more. Lactic acid and urea are excellent humectants that are also keratolytic, decreasing the adherence of dry surface cells, thereby moisturizing in two ways.

Occlusives (like natural lipids) act to decrease TEWL by locking in surface moisture. The most common occlusives are petroleum and animal fats such as lanolin, a mixture of natural sheep oils. Although cruder lanolins that were used in the past often caused irritant reactions, the lanolin used today is more refined and far less irritating, closely resembling natural human secretions. Mink and turtle oils are often promoted. Unfortunately, they are not as good as lanolin, and they will certainly not give you the sheen of mink or the long life of the turtle!

Olive, safflower, corn, wheat germ, palm, almond and sesame oils are examples of unsaturated vegetable oil occlusives (not quite as effective as animal fats). Beeswax and vegetable waxes as well as lecithin and cholesterol are also occlusives. Silicone oils are not only occlusive but are also "filters" which make the skin appear smoother. The problem with all occlusives, especially occlusives containing mineral oil or cocoa butter, is that they often exacerbate acne or irritant reactions. If you have oily skin, you may never need a moisturizer on your face!

There are several high-tech advances in the cosmetic chemistry of moisturizers, particularly in the development of time-release systems such as microencapsulation, nanospheres, liposperes, and liposomes (onion-like spheres – with layers of lipids enclosing layers of water-soluble ingredients – designed to release their moisturizing for up to 12 hours as each layer is sequentially absorbed). New polymers and new forms of hyaluronic acid may also prove to enhance skin moisturization.

There is a bewildering array of moisturizers available. Moisturizers vary not only in their ingredients, but also in the proportion of oil and water they contain. There are two basic formulations: Water-based ("oil-in-water") and oil-based ("water-in- oil"). To recognize the type of moisturizer, dot a small amount on the back of your hand. If it feels cool, it's water-based; if it's warm, it's oil-based. Lotions, gels, and most creams are water-based; ointments are oil-based. "Oil-free" formulations contain synthetic moisturizers in place of natural oils.

For your face

Unlike sunscreen (which everyone absolutely needs), not everyone needs a moisturizer, especially on the face. If you have oily skin, you are often better off without. As a dermatologist, I see many problems stemming from excessive or inappropriate use of moisturizers on the face. If you have an oily complexion but feel you need a moisturizer for non-oily parts of your face, use an oil-free formulation. Everyone should beware of exotic oils, fragrances, protein extracts, or enzymes; rarely useful, they are often irritating.

The most essential quality of a daytime moisturizer is that it contains appropriate sun protectant (see Chapter 4). Products you apply in the day are usually lighter than those used at night. Choose a night moisturizer that will also treat your particular problems such as dry skin, acne, or wrinkles. Chapter 9 will help you decide whether alpha- or beta-hydroxy acids or retinoic acid are for you. If you have no particular problems, you may not need a night moisturizer!

There is no necessity for a specialized "eye cream" – just use the cream you choose for the non-oily areas of your face. If any irritation develops, do not use that cream anywhere on your skin. Your dermatologist could test your sensitivity to the ingredients so you could avoid the specific allergens in the future.

Remember, a moisturizer's price bears no relationship to its performance! Usually less is more; the less expensive formulations are often preferable since they have fewer potentially irritating fragrances and "smoothing agents".

For your body

Body moisturizers can be lotions, creams, mousses, or ointments. Use whichever one you prefer but be sure to apply it immediately after bathing to "seal in" moisture. Thicker formulations are often preferable for the hands, which suffer most from excessive drying. All of the active ingredients discussed in Chapter 9 are appropriate for the body and hands. If you have a problem with cellulite perhaps you should massage the affected areas with a cellulite treatment. These treatments are all moisturizing.

Special face treatments

1 *Steaming* cleanses your skin thoroughly and is especially good for treating oily skin and blackheads; it is not advisable if you flush easily or if you have a very pink complexion with extra blood vessels on your cheeks and nose.

Boil water in a large spaghetti pot with either three tablespoons of Swiss Kriss (a laxative tea) for oily skin, or chamomile tea for regular or dry skin. Remove from the heat. Then put your face at least 8in (20cm) above the pot, draping a bath towel over your head in order to collect the steam near your face. Stay in this posture for about 30 seconds. Repeat if you wish.

2 *Masks* are among the oldest face treatments. Famous women from Cleopatra to Queen Elizabeth had their own special formulas. Masks are essentially exfoliants which remove dry, dead skin cells from the surface and openings of pores, making the skin smoother and the pores less dilated. However, masks do not "nourish" your skin!

Masks can "wash off" or "peel off". The former are made of a clay which hardens as water evaporates. Beware of "natural mud" masks, which can be contaminated with bacteria. "Peel-off" masks contain synthetic polymers that are quite safe and effective. Some masks may irritate your skin; always test a little bit on your inner wrist before you treat your face. If you have oily skin or large pores or if you have dry, flaky skin, application of a mask several times each week can be quite effective. Although many recipes exist for "homemade" masks using natural ingredients, I find them quite messy, and their possible therapeutic effects are minimal.

3 *Astringents* are designed to treat the oily "T-zone" of the face. They are actually "drugs which coagulate protein when applied to the skin surface", thereby constricting surface cells to make pores appear smaller. You know them as toners, fresheners, clarifiers, and pore tighteners, but they all act similarly. Alcohol, aluminium compounds and witch-hazel are the only true astringents.

If you have especially oily areas on your face, I recommend that you wash, exfoliate, then wipe the area with a medicated astringent containing salicylic acid in alcohol and witch-hazel solution. (In general, the higher the alcohol content, the more drying the formulation.) For less oily skin, I recommend pure witch-hazel. Beware of astringents containing potentially irritating ingredients such as camphor, menthol, acetone, sodium borate, or eucalyptus oil. Use them only minimally at first to test your skin for sensitivity.

Special hand treatments

The most common hand problem is dryness! (You learned in Chapter 7 about eczema, irritant dermatitis, and allergies, and about special precautions that you should take if you have these problems.)

For a "quick fix" for dry hands, try the "occlusion treatment" often recommended by dermatologists. Apply plenty of moisturizing cream to your hands. Put on cotton gloves (which can be bought inexpensively in a photographic store), then snug, latex surgical gloves (which can be found at any medical store or chemist). After two hours (or overnight), remove your gloves to see beautifully smooth, moisturized hands!

Perspiration

There are two types of sweat glands (as explained in Chapter 2). The eccrine glands which are most numerous on the palms, soles, and forehead, and the apocrine glands which are in the armpits, anogenital area, nipples, eyelids, ear canal (secreting ear wax) and around the belly button. The apocrine secretions are regulated by sex hormones that activate at puberty and decline with old age. It is the apocrine sweat which breeds the bacteria that causes body odor, explaining why pre-adolescents and the elderly usually suffer less from this problem.

People of African descent have the most sweat glands; Caucasians have fewer; and Orientals have the least. In general, men sweat more from each gland than do women. Faster sweating (as with exercise) yields more concentrated sweat and increased bacteria.

No sweat!

Antiperspirants are drugs which actively decrease sweat. *They* must reduce sweating by 20 percent or more to be deemed effective. Antiperspirants are made of astringent salts (most commonly aluminium chloride or aluminium chlorohydrate). In general, roll-ons are more effective and less irritating than lotions and creams; sticks, liquids and aerosols are the least effective. Although antiperspirants are most commonly used in the armpits, they can also be used to treat moist, sweaty hands. *Deodorants,* by contrast, are not drugs; they merely mask odor with a perfume or by antibacterial action.

If you have a problem with underarm wetness, you should use an antiperspirant regularly, perhaps adding a deodorant when exercising. If you perspire very heavily, your dermatologist might give you a strong, prescription antiperspirant to use daily for a short time, and then several times each week thereafter. Antiperspirants have a cumulative effect; after an initial loading dose, one application decreases sweating for several days!

If you suffer from excessive sweating, your dermatologist might also prescribe *ionophoresis* treatment. This decreases perspiration by transferring ions with a small piece of equipment that can be used either at home or in a dermatologist's office. The ionophoresis apparatus has attachments for armpits, hands and feet to deliver a mild, tingling, non-painful, electrical charge. Seven to ten daily treatments of about 15 minutes each, followed by four weekly treatments, decrease sweating for a period of six to eight weeks.

Ten tips on body odor and sweating

1 Antiperspirants should never be applied to broken, irritated skin, or just after shaving.
2 Stop using your antiperspirant if you feel stinging or itching or if you develop a rash.
3 Apply the antiperspirant only to the armpit or sole, not to the surrounding skin. If it drips down your side, wipe it off.
4 When applying an antiperspirant after washing, be sure the armpits or soles are dry.
5 Antiperspirants are best applied at night.
6 Use a deodorant soap in the armpits, genital area, and feet, but never on your face!
7 Avoid wearing synthetic clothing and especially tight plastic or rubber shoes and boots.
8 After a bath or shower, dust your armpits, soles and all body folds with an absorbent deodorant powder or baking soda.
9 Avoid eating garlic, onions, vinegar, sharp cheese, and mustard, all of which enhance body odor. Avoid hot spices and coffee if they make you sweat more.
10 Shaving the armpits decreases bacteria and therefore body odor.

Tea compress treatment

Just as tannic acid "tans leather", so it can decrease sweating to control moist palms and soles, perspiration under the breasts or unpleasant odor in the groin. Just brew a strong tea using three or four tea bags in 1qt (2.2litres) of water. Cool the tea and either soak your hands or feet, or put some tea on a piece of cotton gauze or a washcloth and apply as a compress to the areas needing treatment, for 20 minutes each day.

Your Personal Skin Care

	Beneficial Cleansers	Special Care and Important Hints
Face		
Sensitivity	- Mild cleansers or soaps - Oatmeal soaps - Avoid perfumed soaps	- Use light, non-scented sunscreen of high SPF - Minimize perfumes, cosmetics, foundations - Avoid retinoic acid
Dryness	- Mild cleansers or soaps - Emollient cleansers (glycerine) - Superfatted soaps	- Avoid excessive washing - Avoid dry environments - Try · - and/or , - hydroxyacids

Flakiness	- Salicylic acid
	- Ketoconazole shampoo
	  (as soap) (prescription only)
		- Your dermatologist may prescribe hydrocortisone
		  or ketoconazole

Large pores Oiliness	- Salicylic acid - Sulfur - Benzoyl peroxide - Avoid superfatted soaps	- Wash at least three times each day - Use astringents - morning and night - before and after exercise - Use masks, preferably in the morning - Facial steaming several times a week - Use non-oily sunscreens (preferably with titanium dioxide) - Avoid liquid foundations - Use dry powder makeups, oil-free cosmetics - Minimize use of moisturizers

Acne	- As for oily skin
	- Cleansers with resorcinol
	  (prescription only)
		- Minimize use of moisturizers
		- Avoid all but gentle exfoliation if you have pustules or cysts
		- Your dermatologist may prescribe topical antibiotics,
		  retinoic acid, resorcinol, or azeleic acid

Extra blood vessels Rosacea	- Sulfur	- Avoid retinoic acid - Avoid steam baths, hot water - Your dermatologist may prescribe metronidazole - Avoid excess alcohol, hot spices, hot caffeine
Wrinkles	- Salicylic acid	- See Chapter 9
Dark spots Mottled pigmentation	- Salicylic acid	- Always apply a high SPF sunscreen - Exfoliate - Your dermatologist may prescribe retinoic acid, hydroquinone, azeleic acid, or kojic acid
Hands		
Dryness Scaliness	- Mild cleansers or soaps	- Minimize washing; avoid harsh commercial brands - Always apply a moisturizer after washing - Try · - and/or , - hydroxyacids - Wear gloves in cold weather! - Occlusive hand treatment
Body, Arms, Legs		
Sensitivity	- Mild cleansers or soaps	
Dryness	- Salicylic acid	- Exfoliate - Apply moisturizer immediately after washing - Minimize washing - Try · - and/or , - hydroxyacids
Sandpaper-like upper arms or lateral thighs Scaly or itchy patches	- Salicylic acid	- Exfoliate - Try · - and/or , - hydroxyacids - Your dermatologist may prescribe retinoic acid
Body odor	- Deodorant cleansers for problem areas	- Use astringents before and after exercise - Apply antiperspirant to armpits - Tea compress treatment
Feet		
Dryness	- Mild cleansers or soaps	- Exfoliate - Occlusive foot treatment
Odor	- Deodorant cleansers or soaps	- Medicated antiperspirant - Foot powder or baking soda - Use astringent before and after exercise - Tea compresses or soaks - Avoid closed plastic and leather shoes

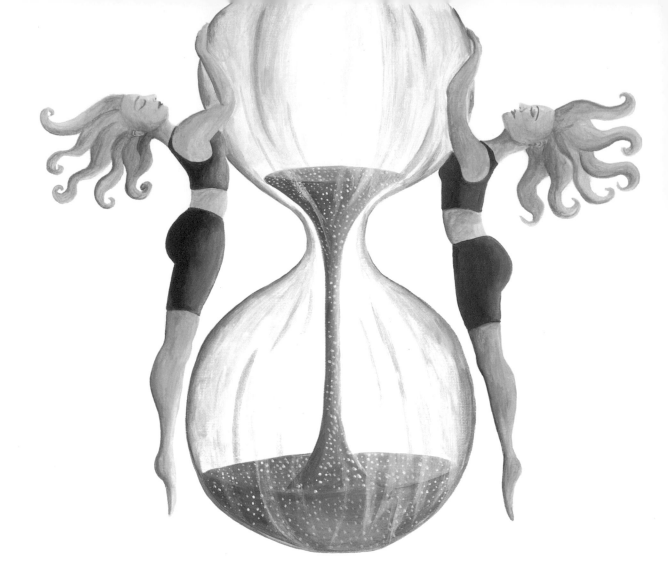

Looking Better Every Year:
What You Can Do

Twentieth-century medical science has practically doubled our expected lifespans, and we are not only adding "years to life" but also "life to years". Those of us in our forties can now expect to live four decades longer than our grandparents (who were in their prime at the turn of the century), and everyone is also enjoying a markedly better quality of life. It is now known that following simple and healthy systems, such as limiting the fat in your diet, exercising regularly and not smoking can prevent, delay or mitigate the debilitating effects of many diseases.

Take heart! It is possible to feel better and better as we grow older. Along with our good health, we can – and should – look as young as we feel!

Our appearance does contribute very profoundly to how we feel about ourselves. There is no doubt that as we see ourselves looking younger, we actually do feel healthier and more energetic. Every doctor knows that one of the first signs of illness or depression is when a person loses interest in his or her looks; conversely, the signal that the same person is getting better is often the renewed attentiveness to appearance. With this in mind, the cosmetics industry in America has launched a *Look Good, Feel Good* campaign, helping hospital patients look better in order to enhance their response to medical treatment. The result is often a shorter recovery time!

Taking care of our appearance, trying to look as young as we feel is neither a vanity nor a luxury – it is essential to our health. One of our main jobs in life, quite possibly our most important responsibility, is one form or another of maintenance. We maintain our homes and our possessions, repairing scratches and dents, and repainting when necessary. So shouldn't there also be a greater interest in maintaining our health, particularly our outward appearance, and, more especially, our skin?

As a result of your interest, curiosity and the drive to read this book, you have at your disposal both the knowledge and the skincare tools that work! This book is your guide. You need not be wealthy; you need not have hours at your disposal each day to devote to your program. You need only be aware of the facts about the many skincare choices available to you. As the 20th century draws to a close, you have moved beyond "hope in a bottle". There is now "science in a bottle" – products and techniques that are truly effective in making skin appear younger!

This chapter explains how to keep your skin looking young and how to prevent and correct those unwanted signs of aging skin. You will learn the fact, and the fantasy, about the famed "fruit acids" (alpha-hydroxy acids), about "retinoic acid" (Retin A), and also about several new products soon to be launched.

Where wrinkles come from? – the six causes

When you take the time to ask "Why?", science will always answer "How". In the case of wrinkles, as you learn *why* they appear, you can also learn how to prevent or postpone their appearance, plus *how* to eliminate many of the wrinkles you already have. It's never too late to care for your skin, to prevent more wrinkles from appearing, and to soften those already present. It's never too late to look and feel younger!

Discovering wrinkles

There are moments in everyone's lives which do not do wonders for morale: among these are the times when you first look in the mirror and notice wrinkles that have made their first appearance. You can ask yourself, am I aging overnight? Am I really getting old? Am I mortal after all?

This frightening discovery can take place when you are 25 years old, or 30, or 40. And inevitably, such moments recur throughout your life with increasing impact, especially as you reach 50 or

60. But It has become clear that these are ages that are all young by today's changing standards – too young to look old! So read on.

The face as a map

Your face is a unique part of your body in that your facial muscles attach directly to the skin rather than to bones or cartilage. There are 120 muscles in your face, responsible for all of the subtle movements that show so much about your thoughts and moods. In fact, humans are unique among living species in communicating so expressively through the face. Although we are told that "the eyes are the mirror of the soul," it is actually the muscles around the eyes that make them so. The tiniest squint can indicate "hidden" laughter, intense thought, or deep anger. But it is not only the eyes that reflect the soul. The slightest pursing of the lips shows emotions as varied as flirtatious invitation or disdain. Furrowing the brow means concentration or reprimand. Tightening the jaw indicates anger or determination. Each of these facial-muscular movements wrinkles your skin, and over time some of these wrinkles become a "permanent" part of your facial "map" – permanent, that is, until they are treated!

What do all these exquisite and exuberant facial expressions do to our facial skin? Put simply, they make wrinkles! These wrinkles have

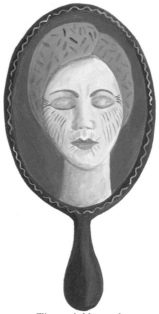

Tiny wrinkles on the skin's surface can be treated at home by exfoliation and creams.

their good side: in the popular terminology they are "character lines". They are a map to your character and your emotions. Without facial wrinkles you would, in fact, be catatonic; you would not have permitted normal and healthy emotional expression. None of us, however, wants too much "character" etched on our face. We feel young, but we do not wish to be a young person trapped in an old appearance. Therefore you need to learn the joys of skincare, and therefore my skin program.

The magic mirror

Your skin is there for all to see. Dermatologists and plastic surgeons carefully observe and classify wrinkles in order to treat them. You can do the same. As you read through this book, look in a mirror in a brightly-lit room to carefully observe telltale wrinkles along with signs of skin damage. Then visit a dermatologist and ask important questions about what you've seen. She or he will be delighted to address problems and recommend solutions.

The six causes

There are six major causes of our facial wrinkles:

1 Natural or "intrinsic" aging

Natural, biologic aging is responsible for the inevitable thinning of our skin accompanied by the loss of structural collagen and elastic tissue, as you learned in Chapter 2. The good news is that this biologic aging is the least important of the causes of wrinkles on your face.

2 Sun damage

The sun is responsible for at least 90 percent of the appearance of skin aging. The sun is the most destructive and also the most preventable of the causes of wrinkles. You learned in Chapter 4 that the sun causes the skin to take on a leathery texture, with permanently etched deep creases. No one wants their face to look and feel like a thickened hide! You can prevent these deep, sun-induced wrinkles by applying a high-protection sunscreen and always wearing a hat.

3 Your facial expressions

While the sun is largely responsible for most of your wrinkles, it is your facial expressions that cause all the furrows that become imprinted on your face. Once again, there is hope! Many of these deep creases are indeed avoidable, and all of them are treatable!

The human face is indeed exquisite in its ability to communicate so profoundly through expression. Indeed, it is remarkable that wrinkling your face thousands of times each day – and hundreds of millions of times in your lifetime – results in so few lasting facial markings. Although most facial movements are essential and attractive, you can learn to avoid or minimize certain nervous habits, such as wrinkling the nose when laughing, wrinkling the forehead to show sincerity or incredulity, or grimacing unnecessarily when watching television. By observing other people's expressions, you can see why their wrinkles and

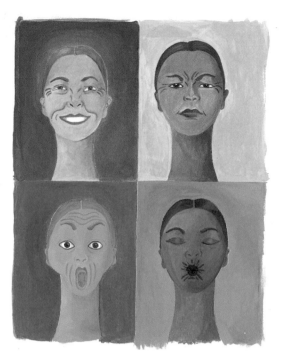

Your expressions can become imprinted on your face as wrinkles and furrows. Avoid unnecessary scowls!

creases form. But how can you recognize your own habits? It's not easy to observe your own face in action. To learn something about your subtle, often unconscious facial movements, you might ask a good friend to observe your habitual facial expressions.

Alternatively, you can keep a mirror near your telephone to observe your own facial expressions as you speak, noting exaggerated or unnecessary movements. If you squint when you read or drive, get glasses. If your eyes are sensitive to the sun, wear sunglasses.

I recall a beautiful 60-year-old patient whose skin looked 80 years old on the right side of her face, and 40 on the left. She had suffered an accident 20 years before, which had immobilized her right forehead. She had a distinct habit of wrinkling her forehead whenever she spoke, prematurely aging the left side of her face which retained its movement.

Although some European surgeons actually operate on a patient's nerves in order to preclude wrinkling of the forehead, I do not advocate this treatment myself. More recently, a new treatment has been developed (see Chapter 10), which involves injecting into the forehead a carefully controlled dosage of a paralyzing toxin that has been used for years to cure muscular spasms or tics, in order to temporarily (for several months) block wrinkling. This treatment often has the additional benefit of breaking the habit of unnecessarily wrinkling the forehead.

Facial expressions are a matter of habit – but they can be changed without too much difficulty. If you notice that you wrinkle your face frequently and unnecessarily, you can break the habit. Simply place a small piece of medical tape (or the sticky part of a plaster or Band-Aid) across your wrinkles when you are alone to become aware of habitual movements you can avoid.

One very important point is that you should *not* try to become expressionless! Everyone looks better and communicates better when they show their feelings. Your face *should* have personality and character. I always recommend a smile! In your daily life, I hope that you smile often. It takes only half as many muscles to smile as it does to frown! If you don't have *any* wrinkles at all, you obviously haven't laughed enough during your life!

4 Gravity

The whole universe is held together by gravity. The movements of the earth around the sun (determining the seasons) and of the moon around the earth (regulating the tides) are all according to the invisible force of gravity. Although gravity makes life possible (and helps people walk rather than float!), we are not often conscious of gravity's effect on our appearance.

But gravity does affect how we look. Gravity probably contributes to the gradual elongation of our earlobes and nose. And as we age, gravity pulls our skin down! With the natural thinning of our skin with age and loss of underlying fat comes drooping, especially of the eyelids and jowls.

Resorption (or shrinking) of bone usually accelerates as we reach our late 50s or early 60s. Especially prominent can be the regression of the jawbone and cheek bones, which in turn contribute to sagging jowls. If we lose teeth and dentures are needed, the bony ridges that usually hold our teeth can erode. Our lips can contract, and wrinkles appear. Gravity exacerbates the effects of all of these natural changes.

Another cause of gravity-induced wrinkles is major weight loss. If you allow yourself to become overweight or obese, your skin has no choice but to stretch to accommodate. As you (hopefully) lose that extra weight, you may suffer not only from stretch marks, but also from having excess skin! The younger you are, the more resilient is your skin. When a younger person loses weight, the skin reforms to a thinner body; with age, excess skin just droops.

The key to retarding this immutable force of gravity on your skin is *prevention*. Do not let yourself become overweight. Always exercise to protect your muscles and bones. Eat a healthy diet to provide your system with essential supplements. Take good care of your teeth to avoid the need for dentures. You will not only enjoy a longer life in better health, but also a better, more youthful skin with fewer wrinkles.

5 Your sleeping position

The average person sleeps for one-quarter to one-third of his or her life. By the time you reach 60 years old, you will have slept for 15–20 years! What you may not be aware of is that while you have been sleeping, you have spent 6–8 hours each day pressing wrinkles into your face!

A dermatologist or plastic surgeon can almost always recognize the side on which you tend to sleep because your wrinkles are deeper on that side. If you sleep with your arm over your face, you may actually be pushing extra wrinkles into one side of your face. If you have diagonal wrinkles across your forehead or cheeks (running from your temples to the mid-forehead or from your cheekbones inward), these lines are not from your facial expressions but from your sleeping position. In children these wrinkles disappear as soon as they get out of bed; but in adults, unfortunately, they can become permanent.

Thousands of years ago, Chinese women recognized that they could prevent creases appearing on their faces by sleeping on their backs, using concave porcelain pillows. You don't need to suffer so much to learn not to bury your face in your pillow! You can easily learn to sleep in a different position. If models and actresses can sleep on their backs, face-up to prevent wrinkles, so can you! To develop the habit and to make this position more comfortable, just place a pillow under your knees.

I have two other pieces of simple advice to help you sleep comfortably without adding wrinkles to your face. Firstly, invest in a silky-smooth, satin pillow case: It's luxuriously comfortable, and your skin does not "stick" to satin as it might to cotton, especially if you perspire occasionally. Secondly, use a big, soft, non-synthetic pillow that does not apply added pressure to your facial skin if you tend to toss and turn.

If you become conscious of your sleeping habits, with very little effort you can prevent your time asleep from leaving its mark on your face!

6 Smoking

Cigarette smoking actually accentuates facial wrinkles! You can often immediately recognize long-term cigarette smokers by their wrinkles: smokers in their 40s often have as many facial wrinkles as nonsmokers in their 60s. Particularly prominent in smokers are tiny wrinkles spreading from the upper and lower lips (especially noticeable in women, as lipstick runs into them).

Crow's feet are more accentuated in smokers. Also, deep lines and numerous shallow lines form on a smoker's cheeks and lower jaw. Often, the cheeks are slightly hollow, probably from the muscular motion of inhaling. A smoker's facial skin often looks leathery and gray because nicotine constricts small blood vessels.

I urge you *stop smoking now*. In addition to all of the health problems and complications caused

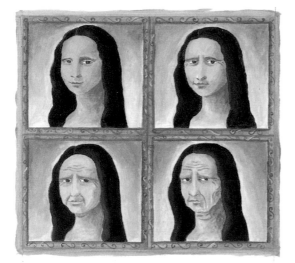

When da Vinci painted Mona Lisa, she had few creases; by her 40s, 50s and 60s, she would have been a different picture!

by cigarettes, if you smoke, you will not look as good as you might, and your skin will inevitably suffer considerable damage.

How to eliminate wrinkles

Some wrinkles are superficial; some can be deeper. The good news is that, as a scientist and a dermatologist, I can assure you that *almost* all wrinkles can be either prevented, or at least successfully treated!

How do you make your skin, and therefore yourself, look better and younger without expending a great deal of time and effort? Of course you can *prevent* new wrinkles from forming, starting today! But once wrinkles are in place, you can add to your health regime successively, as needed, one of three methods to eliminate them – the *"three R's"* – *Resurfacing, Recontouring* and *Redraping*. The result will be a fresher, happier, more youthful-looking you.

Prevention

The first and the easiest skincare step you can take is the prevention of wrinkles.

- Protect your skin from the sun (Chapter 4).
- Eliminate unnecessary facial expressions.
- Sleep in a position that does not engrave wrinkles on your face.
- Stop smoking.

Incorporate these simple and effective preventive habits into your daily life, starting now.

But how can we change the past? Nearly everyone has been exposed to the sun. Many of us used to smoke. And we all experience (to varying degrees depending on our genetics and our state of health) natural, biologic aging and later the inevitable tug of gravity. We therefore need to to be aware of the next three stages of care. To effectively treat and maintain our skin and to eliminate the wrinkles we already have, we can add each of these *three R's* to our health regime, successively in life as we require them.

Resurfacing

Resurfacing affects the texture of skin and eliminates the tiny surface wrinkles. Most of these small wrinkles can be treated at home quite easily and effectively.

By learning proper methods of skin cleansing and exfoliating, you can rejuvenate your appearance each day. Wrinkles from previous sun exposure or smoking can be corrected under the care of a dermatologist with creams, such as products with alpha-hydroxy acids or retinoic acid (Retin A). These resurfacing methods and others will be discussed later on in this chapter.

Some people require more skin resurfacing

than can be accomplished at home. People in this position would benefit enormously from medical treatments performed by a dermatologist or plastic surgeon, such as soft tissue implants, chemical peels, dermabrasion, or laser resurfacing (see Chapter 10).

Recontouring

Recontouring eliminates the deep wrinkles of facial expression such as horizontal forehead wrinkles, the crease between the eyebrows (from furrowing the brow), the little lines above and below the lips and around the eyes, as well as the deep, vertical creases above and below the mouth. Recontouring can only be accomplished with medical treatments by a dermatologist or plastic surgeon. In Chapter 10, you will learn when implantation of collagen or of other soft tissue implants and other recontouring techniques might help.

Redraping

Redraping eliminates the surplus, sagging skin of baggy eyes or jowls. Redraping can be accomplished by a variety of effective surgical methods such as an eye tuck (or blephoplasty), liposuction of the chin, a forehead lift or a full face-lift, all of which are performed by a plastic surgeon.

Exfoliation: Resurfacing your skin by manual abrasion

When you refinish a piece of fine furniture, you often sweep off the old surface to reveal the quality of the fresh wood below. Similarly, one of the simplest and most effective methods of eliminating tiny wrinkles is to "sand" the surface of

the skin mildly with a gently abrasive sponge or product. Particularly likely to respond to such treatment are the tiny wrinkles around the mouth and eyes. This mild abrasion mechanically removes some of the dead outer layers of skin cells so the skin does appear smoother.

Polishing pads

A very effective exfoliation of your skin can be achieved by using a specially designed, mildly abrasive pad to gently remove the skin's dead outer layer. I recommend that you use a *Longévité®* Polishing Pad or an Extra-Soft Buf-Puf. If your skin is very sensitive, a terrycloth face cloth is fine. Apply your cleanser to the pad, then rub the pad onto the surface of your face gently, with firm, upward, outward strokes, perpendicular to the direction of your wrinkles.

This is a delicate job: *buff* your face; do not *scour* it. It is fine to rub under your eyes where tiny wrinkles can form, and don't forget your neck! Rinse your face with warm water then cool water, again using upward, outward strokes with either your hands or your exfoliating pad. Do not exfoliate irritated or broken skin.

To save yourself time, exfoliate when you are in the shower or the bath. Alternatively, you might prefer from time to time to massage your face with the dry pad before or after washing in order to attain the benefits of a somewhat stronger mechanical exfoliation.

Exfoliant products

In conjunction with your regular polishing pad, you can also use one of many exfoliating cleansers or creams. I recommend a gentle product for sensitive skin such as *Longévité®* Exfoliant, a waxy cream that gently removes the dead surface skin cells. Simply apply a small amount to areas with wrinkles, and rub with upward, outward strokes against the direction of the wrinkles. The dead surface skin cells wash away as you rinse, leaving your face smoother with far fewer wrinkles.

There are also many grainy exfoliants on the market. But be careful when using any exfoliant with sandlike grains. Keep the product away from your eyes so that abrasive particles do not get into your eyes. If a grain enters your eye, consult an ophthalmologist immediately since it could scrape your cornea.

I also advise you to be careful of exfoliants made of so-called "natural" products. As you learned in Chapter 7, some "natural" components can cause skin allergies or irritations.

Also available are a number of exfoliating cleansers composed of so-called "keratolytic agents" that unglue dead surface skin cells (keratinocytes) to expose the underlying, smoother skin. The most effective of such cleansers contain either alpha-hydroxy acids (about which you will read later) or, even better, beta-hydroxy acids (salicylic acid or citric acid).

Exfoliation does help

Exfoliation effectively resurfaces skin and yields the fastest improvement. Since, as you learned in Chapter 2, your skin forms a new layer each day, you must exfoliate daily to enjoy and maintain the appearance of fewer facial wrinkles. But important as this technique is to a good skincare program, exfoliation only helps the skin's surface appearance. For sun-damaged skin, other resurfacing methods are necessary.

Topical creams: Resurfacing your skin "from the outside in"

Throughout recorded history, medicine men, witch doctors, assorted gurus, and more recently, cosmetologists, have been searching for the "fountain of youth". Today, we are assailed by advertising for mud packs, masks, gels, creams, lotions, moisturizers, treatments and many, many cosmetics that claim to make skin appear younger. How are we supposed to make head or tail of all these conflicting claims?

At best, some of the mud packs and masks exfoliate to smooth the surface of the skin, and some of the expensive moisturizers do disguise wrinkles for a few minutes to several hours. The so-called "moisturizers" hide small wrinkles by transiently covering the skin's surface and by temporarily increasing the water content of the dead, surface skin-cells.

This effect is, unfortunately, short-lived. Because the human body is warmer than the surrounding environment (which is usually quite dry, especially indoors), any moisture that is applied to the surface of the skin soon evaporates, leaving the skin *drier* and *more wrinkled* than it was before. So the consumer, in response, applies even more moisturizer to gain another few hours of reprieve, much to the joy of the cosmetics industry, but not to any real benefit to the skin.

There is , however, also some good news. Medical science has now discovered several compounds that truly repair skin prematurely aged by the sun: retinoic acid, alpha- and beta-hydroxy acids, L-selenomethionine, and natural vitamin E.

Retinoic acid

Vitamin A and polar bear livers

The roots of retinoic acid date to the discovery of vitamin A in the early 1900s. Everybody has a daily requirement of 5000 units of Vitamin A, which is easily attained by eating green and yellow vegetables. A deficiency of Vitamin A causes impaired vision with retinal damage (hence the name retinol), and dry, red, flaky skin.

By the 1930s, high doses of vitamin A were used to treat scaly diseases of the skin. It was found, however, that high doses of the vitamin given for more than several months resulted in adverse reactions, including headache, ringing in the ears, chapped lips, bone and joint pain, hair loss, and, if continued for long periods of time, liver damage. These symptoms of toxicity had already been experienced by Arctic explorers who ate polar bear livers, containing 600,000 units of vitamin A per ounce! The native Eskimos knew enough to avoid this food! Although skin therapy with natural vitamin A was highly effective, its use was severely limited by its toxicity. Other forms of vitamin A were therefore investigated and synthesized. Several synthetic derivatives have proven to be excellent oral medications: isotretenoin (Accutane), first approved in the

United States in the early 1980s to treat cystic acne; and etretinate, first released in Great Britain in the late 1980s to treat serious scaling diseases of the skin such as severe psoriasis. Because these medications could induce serious side effects if not monitored carefully, dosage and patient-reaction must be followed very closely by a doctor.

Unlike these synthetic derivatives of vitamin A, retinoic acid is a natural metabolite of vitamin A – in fact, retinoic acid is the principal form of vitamin A found in the skin. In contrast to vitamin A itself, which when applied to the skin is totally ineffective (because the skin cannot metabolize it as does the liver), retinoic acid (also called tretinoin) was found to be extremely effective when applied as a cream.

By the late 1960s, Dr Albert Kligman of the University of Pennsylvania in Philadelphia had submitted a patent application for the use of retinoic acid cream to treat acne. Retin A (the brand name) became, and still is, the most frequently prescribed medication for acne.

It took more than 15 years for dermatologists to realize that retinoic acid cream does, in fact, also decrease the appearance of wrinkles. This observation was first made not by doctors, but by patients who had, themselves, used retinoic acid for extended periods as acne treatment. Scientific study then substantiated this discovery, proving that indeed retinoic acid reverses photoaging – the skin's premature aging due to sun exposure.

Retinoic acid and wrinkles

As you learned in Chapter 4, the effects of the sun can be seen on the skin of any present or former sun-worshipper in the form of wrinkles, dark spots, roughness, leathery skin texture and a sallow complexion, often with prominent bursts of blood vessels. Under the microscope this shows up as thickening of the outer layer of the skin, with extra grouped pigment cells, and in the deeper dermis, clumps of non-functional elastic tissue and loss of collagen.

All of these effects of photoaging are corrected by using retinoic acid cream or gel regularly for several months. Wrinkles decrease; dark spots fade; rough spots become red and irritated at first but then disappear (unless they are serious precancers or cancers); the skin becomes smoother, the complexion rosy (sometimes even shiny). The skin truly appears younger, not only to an observer, but also under microscopic examination: the outer layer of the skin is thinner; pigment cells are distributed evenly; there is less clumping of elastic tissue, and there is also regeneration of collagen!

However, these advantages are not without their price. The most common problem encountered with use of topically applied retinoic acid is dry, red, flaky skin – especially when first applied. Some people cannot use Retin A, even at a low concentration, because this reaction is so severe.

Retin A also increases the skin's sensitivity to the sun. The user must use a high SPF sunscreen always, even with minimal sun exposure. The irony is that although topical retinoic acid corrects sun damage, if you do go into the sun unprotected by clothing and a strong sunscreen while using Retin A, you would suffer not only more blistering and severe sunburns, but more eventual photodamage, including the increased risk of skin cancer.

In fact, Retin A treatment makes your skin more sensitive to everything, especially to perfumes and cosmetics. Even products you may have used without problem in the past may sting or cause a rash. And anything that may be sun-sensitizing (see Chapter 4) is even more sensitizing when you are using Retin A. When on topical retinoic acid, it is especially important to use a mild cleanser. If you have facial treatments or waxing, be sure to advise the beautician before your treatment so milder products and lower temperatures will be used. It is advisable to stop using Retin A at least four days before any such treatment. And never go to a tanning salon – especially if you are using Retin A.

How to use retinoic acid

Retin A is a prescription drug: it's powerful stuff! Now that you have learned about its side effects, you can appreciate why it must be used only under a dermatologist's supervision. There are six forms of Retin A: one solution (0.05% concentration), used primarily on the scalp since it is too irritating for the face; two gels (0.01% and 0.025% concentration) which are especially good for oily skin but which can sting or irritate many individuals; and three creams (0.025%, 0.05%, and 0.1% concentration). The lowest concentration cream (0.025%) is most frequently prescribed to correct wrinkles; it is as effective as higher concentrations in treating photoaging, and is far less irritating.

To be effective in correcting wrinkles, Retin A must be used every night for at least two to six months. Under a doctor's supervision, apply Retin A at night at least ten minutes after washing with a mild cleanser. You need apply only a pea-sized amount; dab a small amount of cream into all areas of your face, then distribute.

When first used, Retin A can frequently cause flakiness and redness; in such cases your dermatologist will probably recommend that you use it every second or third night instead of daily. You might apply it with a toothpick or a fine lipstick brush directly onto your wrinkles on days you do not apply it to your whole face. It is *extremely important* to consult your dermatologist if you have any acne flares or irritations, and until you establish the preparation and application schedule correct for your individual skin.

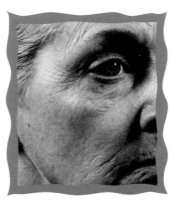

This 53-year-old hairstylist has fine lines and wrinkles.

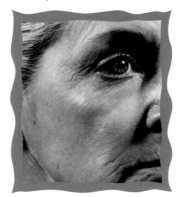

After six months' treatment with Retin A, her skin improved dramatically.
Ortho Pharmaceutical Corporation, N.J.

The conclusion

To sum up, Retin A works, but using it can be expensive. For retinoic acid to be effective, it must be used regularly. Just as you brush your teeth each day, you must daily apply topical retinoic acid, along with sun protection, to enjoy its proven effect on your skin. Retin A is a powerful, prescription medicine that has been proven to treat acne and to reverse the effects of the skin's photoaging. Due to its side-effects, it must be used only under the supervision of a dermatologist. A note of caution: there are no other forms of vitamin A that have as yet been proven to be effective. Do not be fooled, therefore, by imitators: creams advertising "retinol" or "retinyl compound" just do not work!

However, there are other topical preparations that are also truly effective in making your skin appear younger. For advice on these, read on!

Alpha-hydroxy acids
AHAs to the rescue!

Alpha-hydroxy acids (AHAs) are far from new. They have been used for centuries to improve the appearance of the skin. Cleopatra was the first woman on record as routinely applying AHAs. She travelled with a herd of goats to bathe in their milk, which contains lactic acid. Another famous beauty, Queen Marie Antoinette, washed with red wine, benefiting from its tartaric acid.

Technically speaking, AHAs are a group of chemicals consisting of organic carboxylic acids in which a hydroxy group is at the alpha position. Members of this group include: glycolic, lactic, citric, malic, mandelic and tartaric acids. Glycolic acid is derived from sugar cane; lactic acid is derived from fermented milk, honey, and mangoes; citric acid is found in citrus fruits, such as oranges and lemons; malic acid is found in unripened apples and pears; mandelic acid is an extract of bitter almonds; and tartaric acid is found in fermented grapes and wine. These acids are now produced synthetically for cosmetic use. Interestingly, the synthetic forms are less irritating than the natural forms, except for honey extract which may contain a natural soothing agent that reduces the irritating potential of AHAs.

The concept of using AHAs in treating the skin was resurrected in 1974 by Eugene T. Van Scott, MD, and Rueg J. Yu, Ph.D. They realized that AHAs were excellent for treating very dry skin and dry skin diseases such as eczema, keratosis pilaris (a common condition of rough skin on the upper arms, thighs and buttocks that stems from the blocking of hair follicles by excess dead skin cells), psoriasis and ichthyosis (extremely dry skin, which is sometimes called "fish skin" or "alligator skin").

The first AHA cream available on prescription

Table 1

Treatment of wrinkles

with Topical Tretinoin (Retin A) (to be Doctor-supervised)

- Daily or every other day, at least 10 minutes after washing, apply:
0.025% or 0.05% cream to whole face, dorsum of hands, and forearms;

or

0.025% or 0.01% gel to oily areas (especially forehead, nose, and chin); and
0.025% or 0.05% cream to the other areas.

- On days when not applying cream or gel to whole face:
Carefully work 0.1% cream into wrinkles or facial scars with toothpick or lipstick brush.

was Lachydrin (12% lactic acid), still a mainstay for the treatment of these diseases of dry skin. Soon investigations demonstrated that other AHAs, especially glycolic acid, were effective not only for dry skin, but also for treating acne and smoothing wrinkles.

Alpha-hydroxy acids work by helping to shed the extra layers of dead cells from the skin's surface. AHAs not only soften the "physiologic glue" that holds the surface skin cells together, but also inhibit the synthesis of this "glue". As a consequence, dead cells fall away and the skin is left much smoother, both in appearance and in texture. This exfoliation of the surface skin cells also stimulates the enhanced renewal of cells, resulting in faster cell turnover – another indication that the skin is becoming "younger".

Recent evidence suggests that AHAs may act not only on the surface of the skin, but also on the production of "ground substance" – the water-binding molecules in the deeper dermis that you learned in Chapter 2 are so important to healthy skin.

Why AHAs now?

Why the recent explosion in the availability of products containing AHAs? The timing of this phenomenon may well be more commercially than scientifically driven. After all, the fact that AHAs help many skin conditions has been undisputed by dermatologists for more than 20 years.

Here's the inside story: firstly, because the patent for AHA use recently expired, licensing agreements are no longer required so many companies were freed to jump on the bandwagon, marketing various AHA formulations.

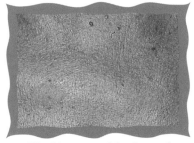

The skin texture of the chest and neck is in need of treatment.

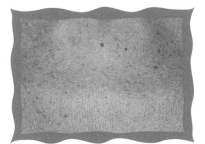

It improves dramatically after three months' daily treatment with Avon's Anew Perfecting Complex containing glycolic acid.
Avon Products Inc., New York

Secondly, AHAs in low concentrations have been officially classified as "cosmetics" which change only the appearance of the skin's surface, not the structure of connective tissue. This classification has advantages and disadvantages: the advantage is that cosmetics may be sold without a doctor's prescription. The disadvantage is that actual proof of the promises on the label of a cosmetic is not required. Not all AHA preparations are effective, so I share with you below my own experience and advice on how to choose the best AHA formulation for your skin.

How to choose and use AHAs

Does the performance of alpha-hydroxy acids match the promise? Yes, when formulated correctly, AHAs do indeed exfoliate the outer layers of skin to treat clogged pores and blackheads, to smooth fine wrinkles, and to remove dry surface skin. You, the consumer, however, are confronted with advertising for a myriad of products containing AHAs, all promising youthful, wrinkle-free skin. Not all preparations are effective. When choosing, there are three key factors to consider:

• First is the *form* of alpha-hydroxy acid: glycolic acid and lactic acid are the most effective for decreasing wrinkles and treating dry skin.

• Second is the *concentration* of the AHA: the higher the concentration, the more effective the AHA. However, higher concentrations can sometimes result in dry, flaky skin and rashes. Concentrations from 1% to 8% glycolic acid and 1% to 5% lactic acid are available without prescription in the United States. These are usually fine provided they are not applied to irritated or damaged skin. Concentrations of 8% to 12% glycolic and lactic acids are available only by prescription since they can cause irritation to your skin.

• Third, is the *acidity* of the particular preparation: in order to be effective, the cream or gel containing the AHA must be acidic. Many formulations, however, are neutral in acidity (pH) and therefore completely ineffective. You can test the pH of any AHA product with litmus paper, which is available from a pharmacy. (This paper, when touched by a liquid or cream, turns a specific color for each degree of that liquid's acidity.) By noting this color, you can determine the acidity of the AHA cream. AHA products are most effective at an acidic pH of 3 or below. (Neutral pH is 7; something is "acidic" if the pH is lower and "basic" if the pH is higher. The surface of the skin is slightly acidic, at a pH of 5.5.)
AHAs can be applied to your face once or twice each day when treating wrinkles. If you use a

prescription formulation, follow your doctor's advice. If treating very dry skin, 12% lactic acid is often prescribed by your dermatologist to be used three or four times each day.

Take care with AHAs

Without doubt, the effect of alpha-hydroxy acids increases your skin's vulnerability to the sun. If you use AHAs, be careful, and commit yourself to decreasing your exposure to the sun by always applying a sunscreen of SPF greater than 20, always wearing a hat and other cover-ups when outdoors, and minimizing outdoor activities during peak sunlight hours whenever possible.

Another caution is that use of AHAs results in more intense skin penetration by other cosmetics and skin medications, thereby sometimes causing irritation that might not otherwise occur. Changing cosmetics or decreasing your use of AHA will often solve the problem. Consult your dermatologist if you need advice.

Which is better, Retin A or AHAs?

As you have read, both retinoic acid and AHAs decrease wrinkles. Both require more than one or two months to show improvement. And both must be used regularly for continued benefit. Table 2 compares retinoic acid with AHAs. Retinoic acid is somewhat more effective, but it more frequently causes adverse reactions, such as increased sensitivity to the sun or to other skin-care products as well as dry, red, flaky skin, especially when it is first used. That is why Retin A requires a prescription while some AHA creams

Table 2

A comparison of retinoic Acid and AHA's		
	Retinoic acid	AHAs
Correction of wrinkles	*Yes (more effective)*	*Yes (less effective)*
Action on skin	*Superficial and deep*	*Primarily superficial*
Time to see improvement	*2–3 months minimum*	*1-2 months*
USE:		
Choice of product	*Only Retin A*	*Many formulations*
Prescription required	*Yes*	*Some prescription; some not*
Concentration	*Gel: 0.01%, 0.025%*	*Glycolic acid: 8-12%; 1-8%*
	Cream: 0.025%, 0.05%, 0.1%	*Lactic acid: 8-12%, 1-5%*
Schedule of use	*Once every day or every two days*	*Once or twice every day*
SIDE EFFECTS:		
Dry, red, flaky skin	*Frequent*	*Occasional*
Sun sensitivity	*Much more*	*Slightly more*
Sensitivity to other products	*Much more*	*Slightly more*

do not. Retin A works not only on the skin's surface but also in the deeper dermis. The AHAs act mostly on the surface of the skin to smooth wrinkles and to treat dry skin. Retin A can only be used once each day, whereas your doctor might suggest that you apply the AHAs twice or three times each day.

Beta-hydroxy acids

Beta-hydroxy acids (BHAs) have a slightly different structure than the alpha-hydroxy acids: recently it has been shown that one such beta-hydroxy acid, salicylic acid, is even more effective than any alpha-hydroxy acid in dissolving the physiologic glue that attaches the old, dead surface skin cells to your skin: salicylic acid actually exfoliates measurably better than any alpha-hydroxy acid tested and is effective for longer periods of time. While lactic and glycolic acids increase exfoliation markedly for the first one to two weeks of use, their effect slows down after four to eight weeks. Salicylic acid, on the other hand, increases exfoliation for the full eight weeks. (Longer time periods have yet to be studied.) Furthermore, salicylic acid stimulates even greater skin-cell renewal than lactic or glycolic acids, also for longer periods of time.

There are other important advantages to this beta-hydroxy acid. Salicylic acid is less irritating than any of the AHAs: there is less flaking, far less stinging, and less sensitivity to other cosmetics appled with salicylic acid than with lactic or glycolic acid.

Why are BHAs not given the hype of the alpha-hydroxy acids? Possibly because they have been used by dermatologists for years and because

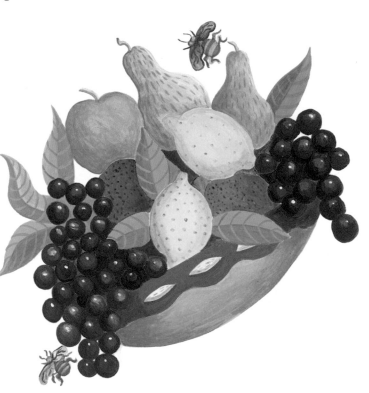

cosmetics companies did not find them as exciting to advertise as the "new, natural fruit acids" (which are not new, and usually not natural).

Free radicals and wrinkles

Everyone is talking about "free radicals", the very reactive molecules that form from exposure either to the sun or to certain cancer-causing agents in the environment. Excessive free radicals damage connective tissue, cell membranes, and the basic genetic building block DNA itself. On the skin free-radical damage causes premature aging and skin cancer.

Because the most common free radicals are made of "reactive oxygen species", the body has evolved an "anti-oxidant defense system" using its own enzymes (often with the help of certain trace minerals) and vitamins drawn from the diet. Being the organ most exposed to the environment, the skin is especially vulnerable to free-radical damage so recent research has concentrated on developing protective skin-cream formulations. Indeed highly effective anti-aging creams containing essential free-radical quenchers such as *selenium* and the natural form of vitamin E have been formulated and will soon be available.

L-selenomethionine

Selenium is a trace mineral essential to human life It has long been known that selenium acts with an anti-oxidant enzyme to quench (or supress) "free radicals".

The natural distribution of selenium throughout the world is uneven. Selenium-rich soils are thought to result from ancient volcanic eruptions with the subsequent leeching to ancient inland seas, long since evaporated. In certain areas, glacial run-off from the Ice Age and wind and rain over the centuries may have washed selenium from the soil into the sea, resulting in a deficiency of this mineral in locally grown plants and animal feed.

Certain areas of the southeast United States, the United Kingdom, the Netherlands, Canada, Switzerland, and the Scandinavian countries have quite low levels of selenium. Some areas (such as South Dakota and parts of China) have such high levels that ruminant animals such as cattle can actually develop metabolic toxicity.

Selenium and health

There is an interesting, important link between selenium and health. In countries where the population consumes more selenium, there are measurably fewer cancers of all types (pulmonary, colon, breast, and prostate, as well

as skin), and in those countries where the population consumes less selenium, there are more cancers. Why is selenium important to our skin? A retrospective study demonstrates that patients whose blood level of selenium is in the lowest 10 percent have 4.4 times the incidence of skin cancer than those in the highest 10 percent. Skin cancers are especially affected by selenium.

The topical cream – a hope for the future

This startling fact led to my own studies, carried out over a number of years, on the possible benefits to our skin of a cream containing L-selenemethionine (which has selenium attached to the natural essential amino acid L-methionine). L-selenemethionine proved to be an excellent compound to deliver selenium effectively to the deep layers of the skin. Using such a cream regularly (or, to an extent, taking selenium orally) not only protects the skin from sunburn (although not as well as a high-SPF sunscreen), but also, in the laboratory, delays the onset and decreases the incidence of skin cancer.

Furthermore, when applied regularly to sundamaged skin, L-selenemethionine cream reverses all of the effects of photoaging better and faster than retinoic acid. Wrinkles decrease and the skin becomes smoother. Under the microscope, the damaged, thickened, outer layer of skin becomes thinner, the clumped elastic tissue is repaired, and there is regeneration of collagen. The still more exciting finding is that this is accomplished without the irritating side-effects of dry flakiness, redness, itching, and increased sensitivity to the sun and to cosmetics.

In fact, L-selenemethionine actually protects the skin from sunburn and decreases skin irritations.

L-selenemethionine cream is not yet available commercially, but it is one of several new preparations that will soon be added to our armament against wrinkles.

Natural vitamin E

One of the most effective anti-oxidants known is vitamin E, a fat-soluble vitamin that can naturally protect cell membranes against free radical damage. Only recently have scientists turned to the systematic study of the benefits of vitamin E to the skin. New research has shown that only pure, natural vitamin E is truly effective when applied to the skin; synthetic forms or derivatives of the vitamin on the other hand, are far weaker. The effective, natural form of vitamin E is called "d-α-tocopherol". Synthetic vitamin E, on the other hand, is a mixture of d,l-α, β,.γ.δ.-tocopherol – 32 molecular forms in all – only one of which, d-α, has full biological activity. Furthermore, vitamin E is often supplied as tocopheryl acetate (oil) or succinate (powder). These forms can be digested in the stomach to form the natural "alcohol" form of tocopherol but cannot be properly utilized by the skin, very much limiting their effectiveness compared to natural vitamin E. Allergy can also be a problem with artificial forms of the vitamin.

One of the only creams on the market containing optimal high concentrations of pure, natural d-α-tocopherol is that made by Longévité®. My own extensive research has proven that this cream is highly effectivce. Just as with L-selenomthionine, instead of causing irritation, dryness and increased sensitivity to the sun and to cosmetics, Longévité®'s d-α-tocopherol creams are designed to soothe irritability and to protect and benefit the skin in important ways.

What about cost?

Very few things are free these days. The treatments I describe above are very effective. They will help keep your skin youthful and repair skin damage, but they can be expensive.

Exfoliation is the least costly of the methods (and the most limited in its effect). Polishing pads are not expensive and well worth the investment since they are designed to provide a safe yet effective level of skin-abrasion. The *Longévité*® Polishing Pad is available in the UK for next to nothing. Beware of more expensive alternatives. Exfoliant products can vary considerably in price. Shop carefully, and see what works for you.

Retin A is good, but it's expensive, enjoying for the time being a dominant market position. A less expensive, less effective, but still good alternative is an alpha-hydroxy or beta-hydroxy acid product. Here you must be particularly wary in view of the wide range of products available, which can vary greatly in price and price is not necessarily an accurate guide to effectiveness.

Looking younger every year

Yes, we can look even younger tomorrow than we look today. We can look as young as we feel. Science is providing us with tools to help our appearance keep step with our longer, more fruitful, more active lives. The best is yet to come!

Nobody's Perfect:
How Your Dermatologist Can Help

If only everyone knew earlier in their lives how to prevent wrinkles and age spots! Fortunately, as learned in Chapter 8, it is also known not only how to slow down those tell-tale signs of aging, but also how to reverse some of the skin damage already suffered, using simple techniques that can be employed every day at home.

Some more difficult skin problems such as acne-scarring, conspicuous blood vessels, and deep wrinkles can only be corrected by a dermatologist. Most treatments that may improve your appearance can be completed in just a few visits to a doctor's office, and such treatments are far less costly than more major plastic surgical procedures (such as facelifts or eyelid surgery).

I must emphasize that I am not recommending any specific treatment or procedure. This can and should only be done by a doctor after very careful examination of the specific circumstances and after thorough consultation with the patient as to the advisability of any particular treatment. It may nevertheless be useful to be aware of some of the widely used medical techniques currently available, all of which can be carried out in the privacy and convenience of a doctor's office. For a few of your dermatologist's "secrets", read on.

Medical miracles?

No, there are no such things as medical miracles. But there are some marvellously effective medical procedures that can help most people look younger! This chapter reveals some of the secrets behind medical techniques scientifically proven to reverse the appearance of aging and to improve other skin problems. It also discusses some of the advantages, limitations, healing times, and expected final results. Anyone concerned with his or her appearance might benefit greatly from understanding these procedures.

A major part of your taking care of yourself, and of your looking as young as you feel, is to be aware of all the helpful technology available. Whether any specific treatment or combination of treatments might help a particular condition and would be advisable in any particular circumstance can only be determined by a doctor or dermatologist after she or he examines your skin problem carefully.

Natural padding
Soft tissue implants

What about laughter lines, forehead wrinkles, or irritating pockmarks? Wrinkles, whether subtle and small or more pronounced (as arise over time from our facial expressions), and indented acne scars or injury scars can all be treated. How? By a recently developed technique, known as soft-tissue implantation, for introducing a safe, natural padding under the skin to even out the surface. Using this simple technique, one of several types of material can be injected by a dermatologist directly into the wrinkle or scar to fill in the indentation.

Such soft-tissue implants have proven very successful in correcting the furrows between the eyebrows, the wrinkles on the forehead, the wrinkles and creases around and below the mouth, and the subtle crow's-feet wrinkles around the eyes. Smoothly indented scars can also be corrected with soft-tissue implants. Only the deep, sharp "ice-pick" scars that result from severe acne cannot be treated by this method.

The collagen system

By far the best and most commonly used material for soft-tissue implantation is injectable collagen. Collagen (as you learned in Chapter 2) is the natural protein material that supports the skin. In fact 90 percent of our skin is made of collagen!

While some expensive mois-turising creams containing collagen advertise that they "rejuvenate" by removing wrinkles, the collagen they contain cannot possibly be absorbed into the skin in a form that would add support and structure to the dermal layer where it naturally occurs. Only implanting collagen (or other implant materials) directly into the dermis can actually correct wrinkles and indented scars.

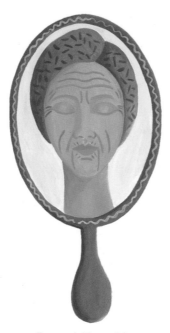

Deep wrinkles and furrows require treatment with soft tissue implants.

longer-lasting and less likely to cause allergic reaction.

Allergic reactions A poten-tial recipient of bovine collagen implant must first be tested for possible allergy to the substance. The test is simple: a small amount of collagen is injected painlessly into the forearm through a tiny needle. The dermatologist examines the area tested a few days later, and again after a month. Almost everyone allergic to collagen shows a reaction within two days – an itchy, red bump appears at the site of the pin-prick. A few people might not show a reac-tion for up to four weeks.

The natural source The actual source of the collagen used for implantation is the same as for so many of our everyday products, the cow. Bovine colla-gen is purified, sterilized, and then treated to remove the small, end-portion of its molecule which differs from human collagen, decreasing the possibility of allergy. The most commonly used form of collagen is called Zyderm, produced by the Collagen Corporation of Palo Alto, Califor-nia. Zyderm collagen has been in use since the 1970s, and was approved for widespread use in the United States by the Federal Drug Adminis-tration (FDA) in 1981. Since then, over one million patients in 28 countries have been treated.

Today, three forms of injectable bovine colla-gen are commonly used: Zyderm I; Zyderm II (Zyderm I at twice the concentration); and Zyplast, a cross-linked form of collagen which is

If you have a history of allergies or of skin sensi-tivity, your dermatologist will probably suggest a second skin test one month after the first to be absolutely certain prior to implantation that you are not allergic. About three percent of those tested have been allergic to bovine collagen.

Would it suit you? Not everyone is a candi-date for collagen. If you have a history of anaphylaxis or of auto-immune disease, you should very carefully discuss collagen injections with your doctor who will probably recommend two skin tests. Anyone allergic to the anesthetic lidocaine cannot have Zyderm or Zyplast colla-gen. And pregnant women are not given any kind of soft tissue implantation.

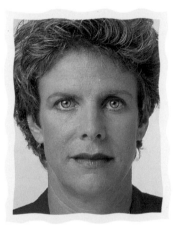

The strengths If a skin test performed with bovine collagen shows no allergy, your dermatologist may determine that you can be treated. The wrinkles best treated by this method are the folds between the eyebrows, which are most prominent in people who habitually furrow their brows or squint, the horizontal wrinkles on the forehead, the deep wrinkles at the sides of the mouth, the horizontal line of the chin (which are always "air-brushed away" in photographs of fashion models), the small wrinkles around the lips, and the crow's feet around the eyes.

A quite popular operation recently has been the use of collagen for lip-enhancement, either to correct the small wrinkles seen particularly in smokers, or to give lips the "voluptuous" look recently popularized by Julia Roberts and other well-known actresses and models.

Bovine collagen implantation is also excellent for the treatment of acne scars. The scars that respond the best are those which are smoothly indented. So-called "ice-pick scars" (which look like large pores) are not usually well corrected with collagen, but can often be treated either by excision or dermabrasion.

Top: before treatment this 40-year-old has prominent wrinkles on her forehead and around her mouth.
Above: implantation with Zyplast collagen has eliminated wrinkles, giving a younger look.
Collagen Biomedical, California

The procedure How is the implant procedure done? Collagen is injected by a dermatologist quite superficially into the skin through a tiny needle. Just after the injection, tiny pinpricks and slightly raised red spots can be seen where the collagen has been placed. (This is because the wrinkle or indented scar is slightly overfilled with each treatment, after which extra saline moisture within the implant material is rapidly absorbed by the system.) The redness and raised spots disappear, usually within hours and almost certainly by the next day. After the injection, the skin surface is then gently massaged.

To enhance the long-term improvement, the patient should try to avoid all facial movements (including speaking, smiling and especially furrowing the brow if those wrinkles were treated) for at least four hours following the procedure. Excessive alcohol and extreme sun exposure should definitely be avoided for at least two days after treatment (as always!). With collagen and other soft tissue implants (unlike more involved cosmetic procedures) the improvement in appearance is absolutely immediate! In almost every case, a collagen recipient can return directly

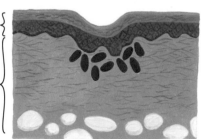

Epidermis {

Thick collagen under scar {

Dermis {

This indented scar requires a collagen implant.

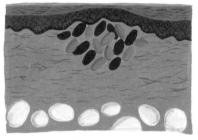

Epidermis {

Collagen implant {

Dermis {

Zyderm or Zyplast bovine collagen is injected at the top of the dermis for correction.

to work and go out on the very evening of the treatment!

Here's how it works Exactly how does the collagen implant work? There are no "tricks" involved: after bovine collagen is implanted just under the skin, it condenses into a soft, cohesive network of fibres (which is the reason for avoiding facial movements just after treatment), filling the unwanted wrinkle or scar.

Over the following months, the bovine implant stimulates the patient's body to form its own natural collagen over the implant. (The implanted collagen acts as a kind of scaffolding over which the patient's cells place their own collagen.) Just as the collagen in everyone's body is constantly degraded and renewed, so the foreign collagen is also degraded, only to be itself renewed by the body's own newly made, natural collagen. The

foreign protein of the bovine collagen is therefore, over the long term, replaced by the body's own natural collagen, rendering the procedure all the more safe. The implant, therefore, offers direct short-term correction (by filling the scar or wrinkle), and indirect long-term correction (by stimulating the body's ongoing formation of natural collagen).

Is the effect permanent? The degree of cosmetic improvement and the duration of the improvement after collagen implantation are highly dependent on the physician's technique. The lasting benefit of each treatment is very individual. If wrinkles are quite deep, several treatments may be required to achieve the best effect. Treatment of indented scars tends to be more lasting than treatment of wrinkles because there is no ongoing force recreating the scar. Facial expressions and sleeping habits on the other hand, can over time reform the wrinkles they have caused.

The long-term correction of such wrinkles can depend on learning not to repeat exaggerated or unnecessary facial expressions such as squinting or wrinkling of the forehead. Remember my advice, though: keep smiling! If you have no wrinkles around your mouth, it means you are not smiling as much as you should!

GoreTex

GoreTex is a synthetic material composed of interconnected fibrils of expanded polytetrafluoroethylene (PTFE). You may recognize GoreTex as the lightweight fabric used to make insulating ski jackets, but GoreTex fibers are even more interesting as surgical implants. They have been used for almost 30 years as surgical vascular grafts and more recently for implants in the skin.

GoreTex patches can be placed just under the skin of the nose to give a smooth profile to previously unaesthetic indentations, and can be threaded under the deep folds between the nose and the mouth to smooth the grooves.

GoreTex is good for enhancing thinned, aging lips, which are often surrounded by wrinkles into which lipstick runs. The procedure is simple and takes only minutes under local anesthetic.

The advantage is that correction is longer-lasting than with collagen. GoreTex is biologically inert and never causes an allergic reaction. If infection occurs or if the correction is not quite what the patient wants, the implant can easily be removed with no long-term consequences.

Fibril

Fibril is another alternative soft tissue material to collagen. It is similar to collagen in the way it is injected, but its composition is quite different. Fibril contains an absorbable sponge of gelatin powder along with a substance called epsilon-aminocaproic acid. When mixed with the patient's own blood plasma and injected immediately into the skin, it causes the fibrinogen protein to form a matrix which fills in the surface indentation of a wrinkle or scar.

Fibril has several limitations: the Fibril procedure is longer and therefore more expensive than bovine collagen implantation because each patient's blood must be drawn to prepare the mixture. Furthermore, the areas treated remain red and swollen for days to weeks after the treatment. And finally, the correction is less long-lasting than in the case of collagen treatment. Fibril, however, remains a possible alternative for people allergic to collagen.

Silicone

Silicone is a synthetic polymer of polydimethylsiloxane which, like GoreTex, has the least physiologic reactivity of any foreign substance ever used for soft tissue implantation. When properly implanted, silicone can be highly effective. Because of complications when it was first used, however, silicone acquired a bad reputation and was eventually prohibited for soft tissue implantation in the United States. Its improved form is effectively used in many other countries.

Getting it right In the early 60s, injectable silicone contained a one percent additive of either oleic acid or sesame oil, purposefully included to enhance the body's reaction to the silicone to delay its absorption and thereby prolong its effectiveness. In some six percent of patients, these additives caused unattractive, red nodules over the site of the implant. These additives were therefore later abandoned.

When silicone was first used, it also had a lighter viscosity, i.e. it was more fluid, with the disadvantage of sometimes migrating between the planes of facial muscles, causing unattractive sagging. Subsequently, silicone of a heavier viscosity was made and found to lock into the tissues much better, with far less possibility of the fluid migrating to other areas. This higher viscosity silicone is now the form that is always used.

A delicate manoeuvre For a successful

cosmetic silicone implantation, the doctor's technique is very important. Silicone must be injected in minute micro-droplets through a tiny syringe (similar to that used for collagen implantation). After injection, the skin is massaged and the patient must not move his or her face for at least 20 minutes. Because silicone is a polymer, which is not absorbed but which remains for ever in the skin, when small wrinkles or scars are treated the indentation is only minimally filled with silicone at each treatment.

The body reacts by creating a capsule of collagen around the implanted silicone with the effect that the tiny particles injected are eventually enlarged by the body's natural reaction. It usually takes two to three silicone treatments spaced at least one month apart to successfully correct deep wrinkles and indented scars.

Silicone is most effective for the correction of the deep furrows around the mouth, the creases between the eyebrows, and for small wrinkles at the border of the lips as well as for shallow, indented scars. Silicone is also the optimal soft tissue implantation material for correction of indentations of the bridge of the nose, particularly after nasal surgery. Silicone cannot be used under the eyes or in deep creases under the mouth or for chin augmentation. It is used only sparingly for treating forehead wrinkles.

Does it work? Silicone, when properly handled, can give permanent correction of scars or indented wrinkles. This advantage is tempered by the possibility that with aging some beading can occur where the skin was injected. The second advantage of silicone is that it is completely inert. There can be no allergic reaction to silicone. In fact, you are already likely to have some silicone in your body! As every syringe needle is coated with silicone, a minute quantity of the substance exists within every person who has ever had a blood test or medical injection.

Fat implantation

Has it ever occurred to you that you have too much fat on your body and too little fat on your face? However, today surgeons are actually taking fat from the stomach or thighs and moving it to the face. The transplantation of fat, or lipotransplantation, is an old and until recently neglected method of treating deep wrinkles, which was revived about ten years ago by the French plastic surgeon, Dr Pierre Fournier.

The actual process In fat implantation, the body's fat is extracted from the abdomen or thigh under local anesthesia, through a small tube used in liposuction surgery. These fat cells, after processing to remove blood and excess fluid, can then be injected into deep wrinkles of the face. The procedure is especially useful for "scowl lines" between the eyebrows, and for deep "smile lines" or folds around the mouth. With lipotransplantation, much more material is implanted than with the other soft tissue implants. For example, only 1 to 2ml of bovine collagen is usually effective for treatment of whole areas of the face, whereas up to 10ml of transplanted fat cells may be required for just two deep wrinkles! Some doctors have also used fat transplantation effectively for treatment of wrinkles of the hands.

Research is currently underway to evaluate the survival of the fat cells transplanted to the face. Some studies suggest that the transplanted fat cells remain in place after one year. Other research indicates that transplanted fat induces the synthesis of collagen over the implant, eventually replacing the implant as in the case of Zyderm and Zyplast collagen.

What are the disadvantages? There are disadvantages to fat implantation: the patient is usually anesthetized or given heavy sedation to undergo the procedure. For this reason lipotransplantation is best carried out with another surgical procedure such as liposuction or a facelift. Also, because of the relatively large volume of fat implanted, the treated areas of the face can appear red and remain quite lumpy for weeks to months after the treatment. Finally, this procedure is usually more expensive than the other methods of soft tissue implantation.

The great advantage of fat transplantation is that tissue from the patient's own body is used to treat the offending wrinkles. The possibility of allergic reaction is therefore eliminated. If someone wishes to correct deep wrinkles and is allergic to collagen, this method is well worth considering.

Hibernating wrinkles!

As you now realize, most of our larger wrinkles are caused by repeated facial expressions: frowning, squinting, smiling, grimacing or raising our eyebrows, or sometimes by moving one side of our face more than the other. With time, our facial wrinkles begin to show our facial habits.

Why hibernation?

You have learned how facial expression lines can be filled and softened by soft tissue injections. You may be surprised that a relatively new procedure actually addresses the cause of the wrinkles by controlling and limiting facial movement.

Through this *hibernation treatment* (as named by one of its inventors, London practitioner and plastic surgeon Mr Dev Basra), a protein is injected to weaken or temporarily paralyze the facial muscles in order to prevent the patient from making unwanted facial expressions. Not only do the facial muscles temporarily "hibernate", but over the period of their hibernation the habit of making certain facial expressions may also be at least partially broken, yielding longer-term benefit.

How does it work?

The material that is injected to induce this static state is botulinum toxin type A (Botox), made for doctors by the Californian company, Allergan. Botulinum toxin was first used in the 1970s by ophthalmologists to weaken very strong eye muscles that caused a child's eye to wander involuntarily. It has also been used over the last few years for treatment of facial spasm.

As with soft tissue implants, the procedure takes only a few minutes and is not painful. The dermatologist or surgeon will ask the patient to frown hard so that he or she can observe the pattern of forehead creases (or to squint if crow's feet wrinkles are to be treated). After injection, the muscles usually start to weaken within two days and are maximally weakened after one or two weeks.

Very occasionally there is only minimal muscle weakening, in which case the treatment may have to be repeated after two to four weeks. The paralysis, or hibernation, of the muscle lasts for about three to four months. After this time, the patient has often broken the habit of moving those muscles that have been treated, so the facial expressions remain softer. Follow-up treatments are also an option.

The body's reaction

Adverse reactions reported after this treatment have been minimal. Although botulinum toxin does indeed weaken or paralyze facial muscles, the effect is only temporary. In rare instances a facial expression with some drooping may temporarily result immediately after the treatment due to the botulinum toxin having set the muscles in an unattractive facial expression. Also, some patients report slight flu-like symptoms lasting for no more than one or two days following the treatment. Patients do become resistant to the drug after about four to six treatments as the body creates an immune reaction to the toxin, rendering it less effective.

Some physicians feel that "hibernation treatment" is an optimal treatment for wrinkles as it treats the cause. Others doctors do not favour it.

Chemical peels

The use of chemicals to "peel away" unwanted or dead skin is a practice with a past. Chemical face peeling can be traced back to ancient Egypt, where creams of alabaster particles suspended in milk and honey were applied to the face for "tightening". The Egyptians also used animal oils mixed with salt and natural minerals, and plant substances to "exfoliate" their faces. Later, poultices containing mustard, sulfur and limestone were used. The Ottoman Turks singed their skin with fire in an attempt to induce light exfoliation (a practice I do not recommend!). In Europe, Hungarian gypsies passed their particular chemical formulae from generation to generation. The American Indians even used urine mixed with pumice for skin application (an unattractive but not ineffective concept!).

The more modern history of skin peeling can be traced back to 1882 when Dr Unna, a German dermatologist, used a mixture of salicylic acid, resorcinol, phenol, and trichloroacetic acid (TCA). British dermatologists began using phenol peels to treat acne scarring in the early 1900s. By World War I, peels were acceptable treatment for gunpowder burns of the face.

The mechanics

A chemical peel involves the application of a substance (usually an acid) to actually burn the surface of the skin to a controlled depth. Cosmetic improvement is attained by the body's natural healing process forming a scar of new collagen. This scar, in turn, increases the thickness of the dermis, providing extra structural support to the skin's surface and a new resistance to wrinkling.

With chemical burning of the skin, there is also destruction of the surface pigment cells and the deeper melanocytes which form the pigmentation. Chemical peels thereby "bleach" the skin to remove dark spots. With healing, the blood supply to the treated skin is also increased, leaving the skin with a rosy glow.

Chemical peels can be divided into three categories, according to their depth:

- Superficial peels – affect the skin only to the bottom of the epidermis.
- Medium peels – affect the skin to the upper part of the dermis.
- Deep peels – burn the skin down as far as the mid-dermis.

The dermatologist selects the appropriate peel according to the type of wrinkles or scars being treated, their location on the face, and the type and sensitivity of the particular individual's skin. The more superficial the peel, the lower the risk of complications, but also the more superficial the correction.

For superficial peels, the most commonly used material is trichloroacetic acid (TCA) in strengths of 10 to 35 percent. Other agents used for many decades are resorcinol and "Jessner's Solution" (which combines resorcinol with salicylic and lactic acids). More recently, formulations of alpha-hydroxy and glycolic acids in concentrations ranging from 50 to 70 percent have been used. Medium peels are performed with higher concentrations of TCA (50 percent). Deep peels are accomplished using phenol or the so-called "Baker-Gordon Formula" (a mixture of phenol and croton oil).

Who is a candidate?

Superficial and medium depth chemical peels can be an effective treatment for fine wrinkles, skin roughness, crow's feet, fine lines around the lips, and uneven, blotchy pigmentation or freckles as well as smoothly indented scars and, sometimes, dark circles under the eyes. "Weather-beaten" faces with pigmented spots and fine wrinkles can respond especially well.

Chemical peels are used not only for cosmetic treatment of wrinkles and mottled pigmentation, but also to treat actinic keratoses (pre-cancerous lesions caused by the sun). The varied skin pigmentation that can result from pregnancy, or from having taken oral contraceptives or hormonal replacement therapy, does not respond predictably to chemical peels.

The best candidates for chemical peeling are women with fair complexions and blond or red hair. Men are not as amenable, with greater chance of scarring following the peel. Patients who suffer from kidney, liver or heart disease, diabetes, and certain scarring tendencies must avoid medium and deep peels.

Prior to considering a peel, the patient should inform the dermatologist of all their allergies or reactions, especially if they have a history of any fever blisters (herpes simplex). Chemical peels have been known to activate fever blisters, so preventative medication must be administered to susceptible people.

Chemical peels cannot improve every skin imperfection. Ice-pick acne scars are not improved, and pores, far from being reduced in size, may appear even larger after a peel. The skin of the neck heals poorly from peeling, often with raised (hypertrophic) scars. Chemical peels, therefore, are done only on the face down as far as the jawbone. Individuals with dark complexions are not good candidates, since the slightest unevenness in the application of the chemical peel substance can cause the appearance on the skin of splotchy pigmentation.

The procedure

Before a chemical peel, the doctor may recommend that the face be "pre-treated" with a special exfoliating cleanser, with retinoic acid, or with alpha-hydroxy acids so that the peel procedure can be performed on a more even skin surface. Just before the peel, the doctor may ask the patient to wash his or her face thoroughly. Then he or she will clean the patient's face extensively with alcohol or acetone, rubbing the superficial oil from the skin.

Chemical peels do sting! The discomfort usually lasts only a few minutes. But these are serious medical procedures. In the case of medium and deep peels, local anesthesia is usually administered. Sometimes in the case of deep peels, tape is wrapped around the face for 24 to 48 hours following the procedure. The patient walks out of the doctor's office looking like a mummy! When the tape is removed the whole face is swollen, and the eyes may be so puffy that they can't be opened for some time. This swelling may last a few days.

The whole face or particular areas can be chemically treated. If the doctor and patient have

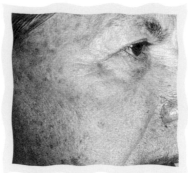

This severely sun-damaged man had many actinic keratoses and very oily skin.

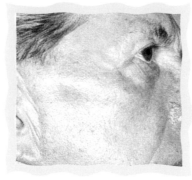

After a medium depth chemical peel, the keratoses were treated and the skin texture was markedly improved.
Chemical Peeling, Harold J. Brody M.D., Mosby-Year Book Inc., St Louis, 1992

chosen to treat only segmented areas, be aware that this can cause a demarcation line or difference in pigment and texture of the skin. A person might show white circles around their eyes or mouth after a chemical peel around those areas.

Recovery

Chemical peeling is not a treatment that yields immediate results. It is rather uncomfortable, and the skin appears extremely unattractive in the healing phase. Superficial peels induce redness of the face lasting several days, followed by flaking of the superficial skin about five to seven days after the peel. For the first week, therefore, the patient actually looks older and more wrinkled than before! Deep peels cause the face to swell considerably which if properly treated should not be cause for alarm. The face will be raw and moist for up to two weeks following the procedure, but the patient must on no account yield to the temptation to tamper with the scabs since that could cause permanent scarring. Your dermatologist will recommend moisturizing creams to soften them.

A light peel takes two to four weeks to heal, a medium peel one to two months, and a deep peel four to six months. It is very important during this healing period not to expose yourself at all to the sun! Sun exposure could cause mottled, dark spotting of the skin. Remember, always wear a sunscreen of SPF 25 to 30, especially if you have ever had a chemical peel.

The risks

Your doctor should advise you of the risks of chemical peeling. Anyone who has ever suffered from a fever blister could, during the healing period after chemical peeling, develop such blisters over the entire area treated. In anticipation of such a problem, the physician might prescribe the anti-viral prescription pill Zovirax (acyclovir) as a preventative. Needless to say, if anyone is contemplating even a light chemical peel, it is important that they advise their doctor if they have ever previously experienced even only one very small fever blister.

The most frequent adverse effect of chemical peels is the minor irregularity in contour between the treated and untreated areas of the skin. This does gradually disappear over time. As mentioned above, mottled, dark spots, or hyper-pigmentation, will result if the peeled skin is exposed to any ultraviolet rays, either from the sun or from tanning beds.

Another possible adverse effect of chemical peels is the loss of pigmentation. If segments of the face are peeled, those areas can appear whiter than the surrounding skin. Uneven depth of peel can also cause some white spots. These white areas are usually permanent, and must be camouflaged with make-up.

On rare occasions, scarring can occur if the peel is applied too deeply or when peeling is done on the neck and the limbs. Also, scarring can result when a full-face peel is done together with surgery to the face or eyelid. A full-face chemical peel should not be done within two months after surgery.

An A-peeling process?

Chemical peeling has never been more effective, and less hazardous, than it is today. Complication rates are quite low and results are more predictable than ever before. Although the art of chemical peeling is an ancient one, new chemicals and refined techniques have generated renewed interest in this procedure.

The process is nevertheless one to be very carefully considered. That young people (aged 30 to 55) have chemical peels, and sometimes multiple ones, is a relatively recent medical phenomenon. Doctors, therefore, will not know with certainty for several decades the possible long-term health effects of multiple peels. It is a fact that chemical peels are actual burns of the face. Since we do know that serious sun-induced skin-damage is more prevalent in areas of previous burns, it seems a reasonable precaution to expect that chemical peels might also make the skin more susceptible to such damage.

If you have ever had a chemical peel, you must consider yourself obligated, therefore, to use a high SPF sunscreen and to protect yourself very assiduously from sun exposure at all times.

Dermabrasion

Dermabrasion is an extreme form of exfoliation (see Chapter 8). For this procedure, the doctor actually uses a rotating wire brush like a sanding instrument to remove the entire outer surface of the skin. The epidermis and the upper portion of the dermis (about one-quarter to one-third of the thickness of your skin) is usually abraded.

The art and science of the process of dermabrasion lie in determining the correct depth of skin to be removed to achieve the desired cosmetic result. Dermabrasion is a safe mechanical process that can be highly effective, especially in resurfacing aging skin.

How does it work?

Dermabrasion is very similar to chemical peels in the kind of correction it offers. The procedure is most commonly used to treat scars, especially those caused by acne or chicken pox. It is also effective for treatment of fine wrinkles of the skin. Just as a chemical peel, it can also be used to treat freckles or brown pigmentation. Also, as with a chemical peel, the improvement is caused by the healing phase. The abraded skin heals with new collagen and elastic tissue formation, generating a kind of smooth scar on the skin's surface which is somewhat "harder" in texture than the original skin. As with chemical peels, dermabrasion is best suited to individuals with light skin.

Dermabrasion is always performed under intra-muscular or intravenous local anesthetic. Immediately afterwards, the treated area is bandaged for at least 24 hours. As with chemical peels, the immediate healing period looks very unattractive, but surprisingly enough it is not painful. When the dressing is removed, the area appears frighteningly red with a great deal of crusting. These scabs are nature's natural dressing while the healing is taking place; they will flake off spontaneously after one to two weeks. Within 10 days, the skin should begin to appear shiny and red. By that time non-photosensitizing makeup with sunscreen can be used to camouflage the healing face. The patient will then feel comfortable about resuming his or her normal social and work activities. The skin will usually be pink and tender for up to six months after the procedure.

Some possible problems

Following the initial scabbing and swelling of the face, when dermabraded skin becomes shiny and red, little whiteheads called *milia* can form. These can very easily be treated by your dermatologist. As with chemical peels, after healing, a demarcation between the area treated and the surrounding untreated skin might also become visible, the dermabraded skin often appearing whiter and shinier even after six months. In such cases, makeup is used to camouflage the area.

Sometimes the dermabraded skin will develop mottled dark spots, a problem that can almost always be prevented by avoiding all direct exposure to sunlight and (of course) to tanning beds. Individuals with dark complexions may develop such dark spots even without exposure to ultraviolet light. On rare occasions, there can be prolonged redness, though this gradually disappears with time.

Laser resurfacing
High-tech

Let's look at a new, "high-tech" method of resurfacing the skin. A laser produces a very thin, high-powered beam of energy that actually

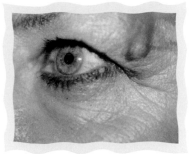

Aged 40, this woman has many tiny wrinkles and crêpe-like skin around the eyes.

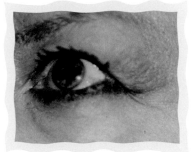

Three months after laser skin resurfacing, her skin is smooth, with barely any wrinkles.
Sharplan Lasers Inc., N.J.

vaporizes the skin's surface tissue to remove surface wrinkles and dark spots. Recently developed lasers can deliver this energy pulse in an incredibly short time – in fact one-two thousandths of a second! The laser's advantages over chemical peeling or dermabrasion are precision and accuracy. The laser can control depth of treatment with great precision. Although previous lasers risked scarring when heat was conducted to secondary skin tissue, modern "ultra-pulse" lasers minimize such risk of thermal burn and so are ideal for eliminating wrinkles on sensitive areas. The surgeon can operate the laser with magnifying instruments, targeting each wrinkle very accurately.

Laser resurfacing can be performed on specific wrinkles and scars, on limited areas of the face, or on the entire face. The method is excellent for dealing with superficial wrinkles and scars but is not effective for deep wrinkles such as those between the eyebrows or the furrows at the side of the mouth (for which implants such as collagen are best). The laser's precision is ideal for people with more pigmented skin as there is less uneven, splotchy pigmentation after healing.

The down-side

There are disadvantages to this high-tech magic. Most significantly, the skin's healing time is longer then for a chemical peel or dermabrasion of comparable depth. After a laser abrasion, there is so much swelling and redness that most patients avoid leaving home for at least ten days. Redness can persist for up to two to three months and, in rare cases, for even longer! After two weeks, it is safe to apply makeup over the affected area. But treatment by laser can increase the skin's sensitivity to many makeups or creams, and anything that irritates the skin must be discontinued.

Other disadvantages are similar to those that occur after chemical peels and dermabrasion: mottled dark spots can appear; a visible line between laser-abraded and untreated skin might show and herpes virus can be activated if preventative medication is not taken. This procedure is usually more expensive than a comparable chemical peel, reflecting the cost of the sophisticated laser equipment.

Your doctor, your partner

As Linus Pauling's book title promised, today you can "live longer and feel better" than ever in history. You can also suit your appearance to your enhanced good health. It's entirely up to you. If you wish to appear as young as you feel, today's medical science has given us effective means. Your doctor can be your partner in this effort.

Index

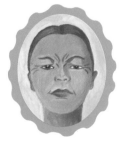

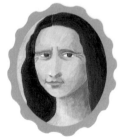

Bibliography

Aging and the Skin, Edited by Arthur K. Balin and Albert M. Kligman, New York, Raven Press, 1989

Thin Thighs for Life, Karen Burke, London, Hamlyn, 1995

Dermatologic Surgery

Dermatology in General Medicine, Edited by Thomas B. Fitzpatrick, Arthur Z. Eisen, Klaus Wolff, et al., New York, McGraw-Hill Book Company, 1987

Cosmetics in Dermatology, Zoe Diana Draelos, New York, Churchill Livingstone, 1995

Contact Dermatitis, Alexander A. Fisher, Philadelphia, Lea & Febiger, 1986

Clinical Dermatology: A Color Guide to Diagnosis and Therapy, Thomas P. Habif, St Louis, The C.V. Mosby Company, 1985

Harry's Cosmetology, Edited by J.B. Wilkinson and R.J. Moore, New York, Chemical Publishing, 1982

Indoor Air Pollution: An Introduction for Health Professionals, Washington DC, US Government Printing Office, 1994

Journal of Clinical Laser Medicine and Surgery

Journal of the American Academy of Dermatology

Dermabrasion and Chemical Peel: A Guide for Facial Plastic Surgeons, E. Gaylon McCollough and Phillip Royal Langsdon, New York, Thieme Medical Publishers, 1988

Dermatology, Samuel L. Moschella, Donald M. Pillsbury, Harry J. Hurley, Philadelphia, W.B. Saunders Co., 1975

Panati's Extraordinary Origins of Everyday Things, Charles Panati, New York, Harper & Row, 1987

Publisher's Acknowledgments

Front cover: "Woman at Indoor Pool" Comstock Photo Library
Author photograph page iv by Manning Gurney
Bridgeman Art Library /National Maritime Museum 13; Harold J. Brody, M.D., *Chemical Peeling*, 1st edition, St Louis, 1992, Mosby-Year Book, Inc. 122 top, 122 bottom; Karen E. Burke Research Foundation 65 top, 66 top, 66 centre, 105 top, 105 bottom, 107 top, 107 bottom, 115 top, 115 bottom, 125 top, 125 bottom; Gloria F. Graham, M.D. 65 bottom; Thomas P. Habif, M.D., *Clinical Dermatology*, St Louis, 1990, Mosby-Year Book, Inc. 66 bottom; Mayo Clinic Health Letter 59 top, 59 bottom; Science Photo Library /Oscar Burriel/Latin Stock 52, /Dr P. Marazzi 43, 63 centre, 64 top, 67 top, 67 centre, /John Radcliffe Hospital 79 top, /St Bartholomew's Hospital 67 bottom, 78 top, /Sheila Terry 75; The Skin Cancer Foundation 63 top, 64 centre, 64 bottom, 65 centre; Nia K. Terezakis, M.D., Clinical Professor of Dermatology, Tulane University School of Medicine and Clinical Associate Professor of Dermatology, Louisiana State University School of Medicine 63 bottom.

Longévité® Skin Care and Cellulite Treatment Products

Researched and formulated by Dr. Karen Burke, Longévité® Skin Care and Cellulite Treatment products are now available. For information on the exclusive Longévité® line, please write to:

Longévité®, c/o Cambertown Ltd, Goldthorpe, Rotherham, South Yorkshire, S63 7BL, United Kingdom. Or telephone or fax Longévité® c/o Cambertown Telephone: 01709 890666 Fax: 01709 897787

If you leave your name and mailing address, we would be pleased to mail to you at no cost or obligation a descriptive leaflet and order form.

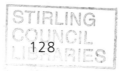